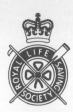

THE ROYAL LIFE SAVING SOCIETY U.K.

Patron: HER MAJESTY THE QUEEN

Incorporated by Royal Charter
Registered Charity No. 279782

SAVING LIFE

THE OFFICIAL
ROYAL LIFE SAVING SOCIETY
GUIDE TO
RESUSCITATION &
FIRST AID

Editor:
Anthony J. Handley, MD,FRCP,FIST

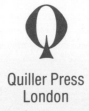

Quiller Press
London

The Handbook

The Society's first Handbook, used throughout the Commonwealth, was published in 1891. This was revised and reprinted on over 40 occasions until, in 1963, branches in the United Kingdom, Canada, Australia and New Zealand published their own handbooks.

RLSS U.K. Handbook

1st EDITION 1963
2nd EDITION 1969
3rd EDITION 1973
The 3rd Edition comprised the main Handbook "Life Saving and Water Safety", "Emergency Resuscitation", "Examiners' Manual" and "On Guard" (the Lifeguard Manual).
4th EDITION 1978
1st Reprint (fully revised) 1984
2nd Reprint (minor revisions) 1985
5th EDITION 1986
1st Reprint (minor revisions) 1989

This book is part of the RLSS Handbook 'Lifesaving', a 7-part volume with a separate ring binder to hold one or more parts. These are listed below and are separately available from local RLSS Branches; a copy of the Society's current "Catalogue" is available on request from RLSS Headquarters (see address below) with price information, etc.

LIFESAVING AND WATER SAFETY: An Introduction

WATER RESCUE SKILLS

TEACHING WATER SAFETY: A Project Approach

RESUSCITATION AND FIRST AID

THE AWARD SCHEMES

LIFEGUARD MANUAL

EXAMINERS GUIDE TO THE AWARD SCHEMES

Preface

The Society endeavours to adopt the same resuscitation procedures as the Resuscitation Council (UK), St John Ambulance, the British Red Cross Society and St Andrew's Ambulance Association. Because advances are continually being made in this field and because respective publication dates punctuate such advances at different intervals, differences between the teaching programmes of the RLSS and other national (and international) guidelines are inevitable. In this text, the masculine includes the feminine and the expression 'lifesaver' includes lifeguards, unless the context specifically requires otherwise. The Society gratefully acknowledges the assistance of the staff of the North East Essex District Health Authority.

This text is published by Quiller Press Ltd., 46 Lillie Road, London SW6 1PN, under the title "Saving Life – the Official Royal Life Saving Society Guide to Resuscitation and First Aid" (1989); it is also published by The Royal Life Saving Society U.K. under the title "Resuscitation and First Aid" 5th Edition, 1st Reprint (with minor revisions) 1989.

It will operate in parallel with the 5th Edition 1986 as a source of information for RLSS U.K. teaching programmes and examinations until 30 June 1989. Thereafter it will supersede the 5th Edition 1986 entirely.

ISBN 1 870948 04 1 "Saving Life"
ISBN 0 907082 31 9 "Resuscitation and First Aid"
ISBN 0 907082 00 9 Complete RLSS U.K. Handbook

Printed in Hong Kong; Designed by Rainbow Graphics, Birmingham.

Contents

1. Emergency Action   5

First Aid
Priorities of a Rescue

2. Anatomy and Physiology   11

The Respiratory System
Lungs
Breathing
Control of Breathing
Blood
Circulation

3. Techniques of Resuscitation   17

Resuscitation
Asphyxia
Cardiac Arrest
Expired Air Resuscitation
External Chest Compression
Sequence of Resuscitation
Summary of Resuscitation
Care of Casualty
Problems during Resuscitation
Special Circumstances
Resuscitation in the Water

4. General First Aid   31

Diagnosis
Minor Bleeding
Choking
Heart Attack
Fractures
Burns
Electric shock
Gas and Smoke inhalation

5. Aquatic First Aid   41

Drowning
Sub-aqua diving
Cramp
Spinal injuries
Epilepsy
Effects of heat
Asthma

6. The Effects of Cold Water Immersion   49

Sudden entry into cold water
Swimming in cold water
Prolonged cold immersion
Body fat
Clothing
Hypothermia
Activity
Alcohol and Hypothermia
Avoiding the dangers of cold water immersion

Glossary   56

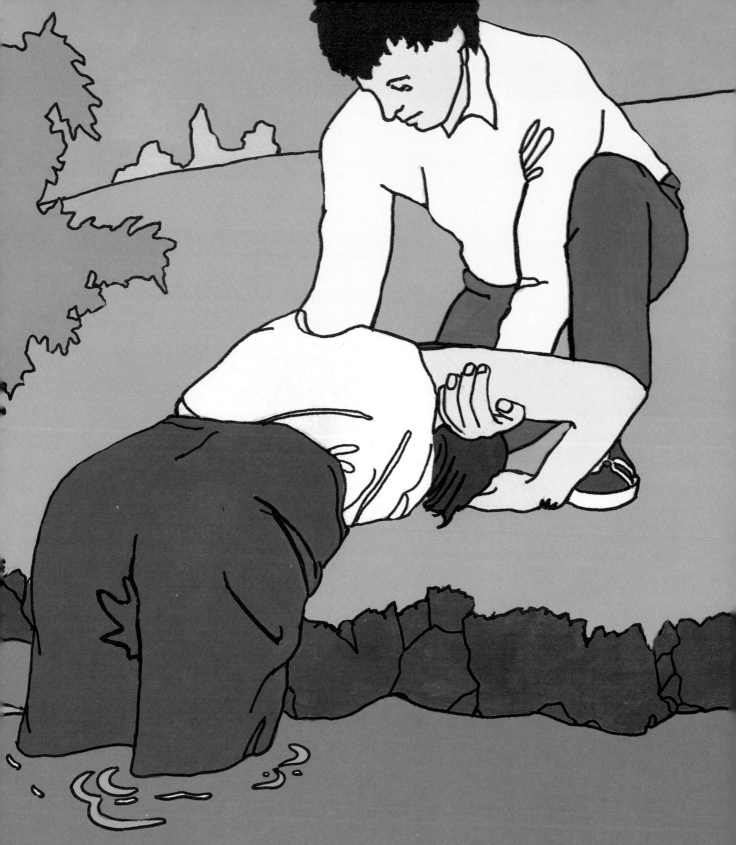

Chapter 1
Emergency Action

First Aid

First Aid is the initial or emergency help given to a casualty before qualified medical assistance is available. From the moment of reaching a casualty until he can be transferred to the care of more skilled or qualified personnel, individual Lifesavers will be responsible for resuscitation and any other First Aid required. Although speed and decisiveness are essential, care must be taken that hasty measures do not worsen the condition of the casualty or endanger the rescuers.

Aims

The aims of First Aid are:
a. To preserve life
b. To minimise the effects of injury
c. To promote recovery
d. To obtain further qualified assistance without delay

Training

To be able to achieve these aims Lifesavers must be well trained and able to assume responsibility for managing casualties. They should have an understanding of the structure and function of the human body and be able to render skilled First Aid, including Cardiopulmonary Resuscitation (CPR).

Through tuition from medical and qualified lay teachers, Lifesavers should obtain recognised qualifications such as the Resuscitation Awards of the Royal Life Saving Society and the First Aid Certificates of the St. John Ambulance, St. Andrew's Ambulance Association or the British Red Cross Society. Thereafter, they should keep up-to-date and improve their basic knowledge and skills.

Priorities of a Rescue

When attending any emergency or incident the would-be rescuer should undertake the following as necessary and in the order given:

- Control
- Safety
- Assessment
- Lifesaving actions
- Care of injuries
- Aftercare and medical attention

Control

On arriving at the scene of the emergency, state that you are a trained Lifeasaver and if there are no doctors, nurses or medically more experienced people present, take charge calmly but firmly.

Spend a few moments collecting your thoughts, assessing the need for safety precautions and gaining an overall impression of the nature of the emergency with which you have to cope.

Safety

Minimise as far as possible the risk of any further harm coming to the casualty, bearing in mind the need for your own safety and that of other rescuers. Where possible remove danger from the casualty, rather than the casualty from danger, for example by controlling road traffic or boating. Occasionally it may be necessary to move the casualty before even the most urgent resuscitation is carried out if, for example, he is in a gas-filled environment.

Assessment

Number of Casualties: By your own observations and by asking bystanders, it is essential early in the rescue to know the number of casualties with which you are dealing, particularly in a water rescue when one or more may have disappeared from sight.

Help Available: The way you plan your First Aid will depend on the number of able-bodied helpers you have available. You may be able to include those who have been involved in the incident once they have been rescued and provided they are not seriously injured or suffering from shock. Determine quickly the capability and training of any potential helpers. Can they swim? Have they been taught First Aid or resuscitation? Do they know the procedure for calling an ambulance?

Priority of Treatment: When more than one casualty is involved in an incident it is important to treat the most seriously affected first. When dealing with an individual casualty, life-threatening conditions must be attended to before less serious injuries and generally in the order given below. (Sometimes however, bleeding may be so severe that it must be stopped before resuscitation can be effective.)

- Cardiopulmonary Resuscitation
- Control of severe bleeding
- Care of the unconscious breathing casualty
- Treatment for shock

The management of these conditions is described below. Attention to other injuries is less urgent and is dealt with in Chapters 4 & 5.

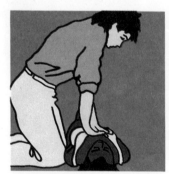

Cardiopulmonary Resuscitation

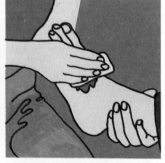

Control of severe bleeding

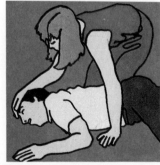

Care of the unconscious breathing casualty

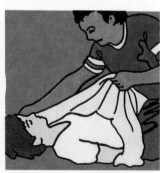

Treatment for shock

Lifesaving Actions

Cardiopulmonary Resuscitation:

If resuscitation is required (External Chest Compression and/or Expired Air Resuscitation) this normally takes absolute priority over any other First Aid measures. Details of the techniques are given in full in Chapter 3. In summary they are as follows:-

1. Check whether casualty is conscious.
2. Check whether casualty is breathing.
3. If unconscious and not breathing: turn him on to his back.
4. Obtain a clear airway.
5. Start Expired Air Resuscitation (EAR) if necessary.
6. Check the casualty's pulse.
7. Start External Chest Compression (ECC) if necessary.
8. Combine EAR and ECC (with an assistant if available).

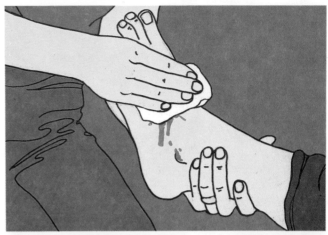

Severe Bleeding

If blood is lost from the circulation, the amount of oxygen that can be carried to the organs and tissues of the body is reduced. If bleeding is severe it can lead to shock or ultimately to death. Bleeding may occur externally (e.g. a cut or graze) or internally (e.g. rupture of the spleen after a blow to the abdomen; bleeding into a muscle after a crush injury). Internal bleeding is difficult to diagnose; signs of shock will occur and the casualty should be treated for this condition (See below). External bleeding is usually obvious but a quick examination of the whole casualty, including any necessary removal of clothing, will ensure that no hidden bleeding is missed.

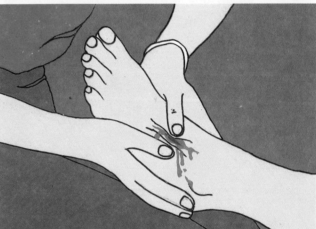

● TREATMENT

1. Apply direct pressure to the wound, preferably using a dressing or pad of clean material; if this is not available use your fingers or the palm of your hand. If the bleeding does not stop, apply more dressings and bandage firmly.
2. If no dressings are available and the wound is extensive, or if an obvious foreign body is present, press the edges together with your fingers. Do this gently but firmly.
3. Lay the casualty down in a comfortable position and raise the injured part if possible. Support it by hand or in a suitable sling.
4. Treat for shock.
5. Summon medical assistance or take the casualty to a doctor or hospital. Even if the wound appears minor, further treatment may be necessary to prevent infection.

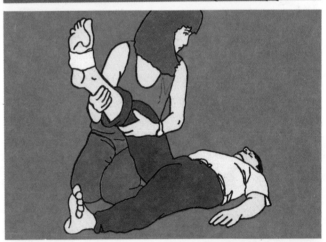

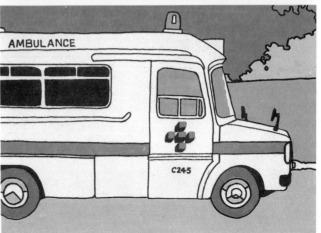

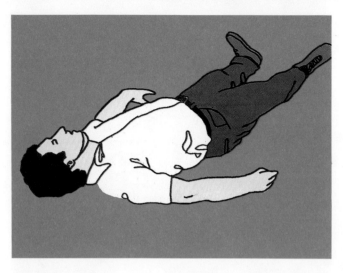

The Unconscious Breathing Casualty

Loss of consciousness results from some interference with the function of the brain due to:

a. A reduced supply of blood: strangulation; heart attack; shock; fainting.

b. Temporary or permanent injury: head injury; stroke; poisoning; hypothermia.

c. Disturbance of the normal electrical activity: epilepsy.

d. A reduced oxygen level in the blood: suffocation; drowning.

e. An abnormal level of sugar in the blood: diabetes.

● DIAGNOSIS

Disturbance of consciousness may vary from slight drowsiness or confusion to deep coma in which the casualty is totally unresponsive. For the purpose of deciding on First Aid treatment a simple distinction between consciousness and unconsciousness can be made by gently shaking the casualty and calling "Are you awake?" "Can you hear me?" Be careful when you do this not to move him unnecessarily as you could aggravate any injuries, particularly of the neck.

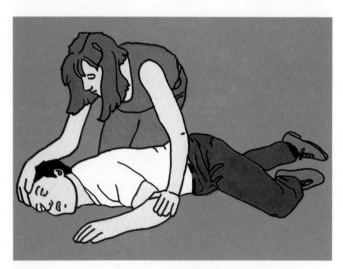

● TREATMENT

1. Remove or treat any obvious cause of the unconsciousness.

2. Ensure that the casualty's airway is clear.

3. Examine him and treat any serious injuries.

4. If he is still unconscious but breathing normally, place him in the Recovery Position (see page 26) unless this would aggravate an injury.

5. Call for further medical help or an ambulance.

6. Keep him protected from cold and wet.

7. Maintain observation of his breathing.

8. DO NOT leave the casualty unattended.

9. DO NOT give him anything to eat or drink.

Shock

Shock can be defined as "failure of the circulation which results in an inadequate supply of blood to vital organs." It occurs when, for a number of reasons, there is not enough blood being pumped round the body. Since one of the main functions of blood is to carry oxygen, failure of the circulation means that essential parts of the body such as the brain, kidneys and heart do not receive as much oxygen as they need and can no longer function properly. Unless the patient is treated quickly and adequately death may result.

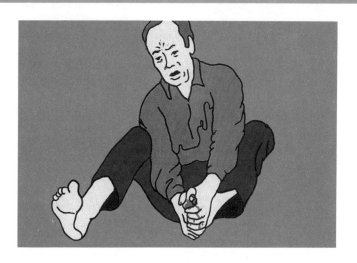

The body tries to compensate for the lack of circulating blood in three ways:

a. By drawing the remaining blood away from the skin and directing it in preference to more important areas.

b. By increasing the rate of breathing to get as much oxygen as possible into the blood.

c. By speeding up the heart to circulate the blood more rapidly.

The signs of shock are produced by lack of oxygen together with the body's compensating mechanisms. The brain suffers most from a reduced blood supply, so that a shocked casualty feels faint, dizzy and confused, and in severe cases may become unconscious. As blood is drawn away from the surface, so the skin becomes pale and cold to the touch. The pulse is rapid but "weak" as the reduced volume of blood in the arteries gives rise to a low blood pressure. Breathing is rapid and the casualty seems to be gasping for air. Sweating often accompanies shock, but does not appear to have any useful purpose, simply being a reflex response to the reduced blood flow.

● CAUSES OF SHOCK

a. Loss of blood volume: external bleeding; internal bleeding; loss of fluid from burns; vomiting; diarrhoea; profuse sweating.

b. Heart failure (failure of the "pump"): heart attack; certain virus infections; severe irregularity of the heartbeat.

c. Other causes: blood infections; severe pain; injury; near-drowning.

It can be seen that the medical meaning of shock has very little to do with the popular use of the word although fear and emotion may make the condition worse.

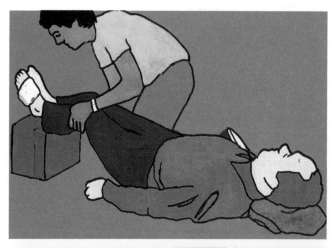

● TREATMENT

1. Treat the cause if possible: stop any external bleeding; dress burns; reassure the casualty.

2. Lay the casualty flat with his legs raised, unless he is unconscious when he should be placed in the Recovery Position.

3. Keep him warm enough to prevent heat loss.

4. Give nothing by mouth because of the possibility that surgery, and hence an anaesthetic, will be needed. If the stomach is full, anaesthesia often produces vomiting and, in the unconscious casualty, inhalation of vomit into the lungs.

5. Get the casualty to hospital as a matter of urgency.

Care of Injuries

The recognition and management of those injuries likely to be encountered by the Lifesaver are described in Chapters 4, 5 and 6.

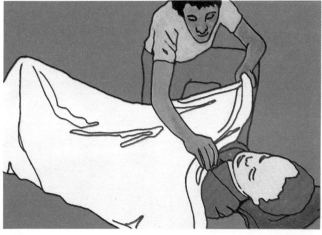

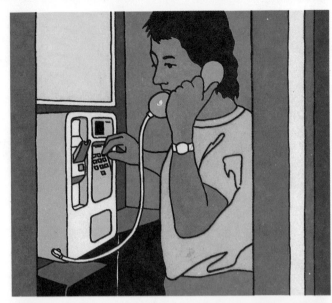

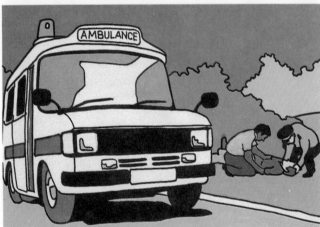

Aftercare and Medical Attention

Unless the injury has been of a very mild nature, medical assistance must be obtained from a doctor or hospital. When in doubt seek advice. ALWAYS obtain a medical opinion if:

a. The casualty has been unconscious.

b. Any resuscitation measures have been necessary.

c. There are any signs of shock.

d. The casualty has been totally submerged under water (i.e. near-drowning).

These rules apply however well the casualty appears to have recovered. After completing First Aid measures, you should obtain medical assistance:

For the seriously injured or unconscious casualty:
by calling an ambulance: Dial 999 from a public or private telephone. Be prepared to give the telephone number from which you are telephoning, the location of the casualty, the nature of his injuries, the urgency with which an ambulance is required and your own name.

For the moderately injured but conscious casualty:
by calling an ambulance or transporting him in a private vehicle to a hospital Accident and Emergency Department.

For the mildly injured casualty or where doubt exists:
by contacting the nearest General Practitioner or taking him to a doctor's surgery.

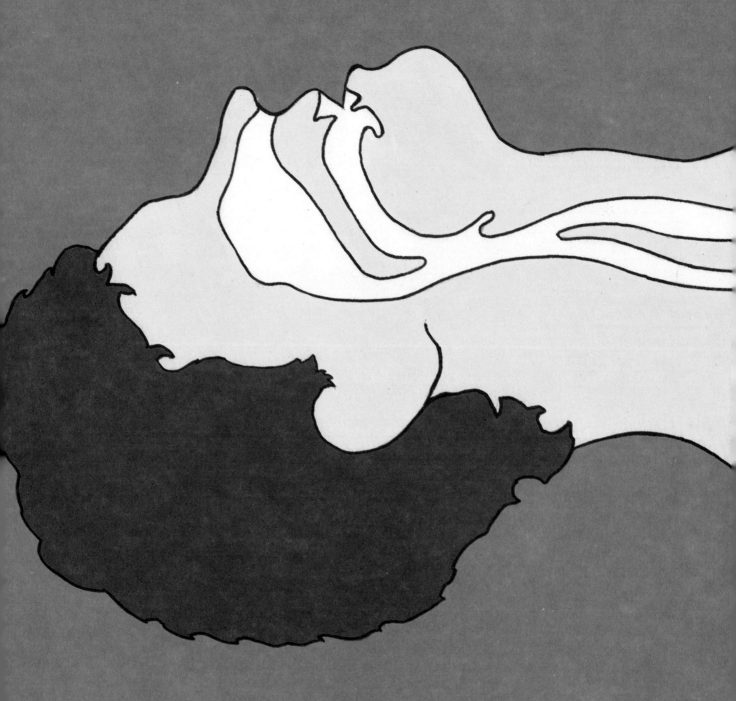

Chapter 2
Anatomy and Physiology

Introduction

A knowledge of those parts of the body concerned with respiration and the circulation of blood is helpful for an understanding of how and why methods of resuscitation are effective. However, it is important to appreciate that the respiratory and circulatory systems are only two of a number of systems within the body that need to work together in harmony to allow us to live and function normally.

The body is built up on a framework (skeleton) of bones which gives it shape and support, and helps to protect various internal organs. To allow us to move, there are muscles connected to the bones either side of a joint. When these muscles shorten (contract) movement occurs. The muscles are controlled by nerve impulses passing down from the brain and through the spinal cord, which lies protected within the bony vertebral column. The nerves themselves travel outwards from the spinal cord and impulses starting in the brain are then able to ensure that purposeful co-ordinated movement takes place.

Energy for muscle activity comes from the food we eat, which is digested (broken down) in the stomach and small intestine and absorbed into the blood. The liver stores the digested food in a form that can be used to produce energy, and is very important also for making harmful substances safe. Unwanted food and other waste products are passed out either through the intestines or in a fluid form via the kidneys. **Oxygen is required as well as food to produce energy. We get this oxygen from the air around us. As we breathe in, air is drawn through the mouth and nose, down the windpipe and into the lungs. Once in the lungs, oxygen can diffuse into the blood; the heart then pumps the oxygenated blood through the arteries to all parts of the body. The brain is the most sensitive part of the body. Within seconds of the heart stopping we lose consciousness due to lack of oxygen, and in a few minutes we die. This is why it is so important to start resuscitation as soon as possible after breathing or the heart has stopped, whatever the cause.**

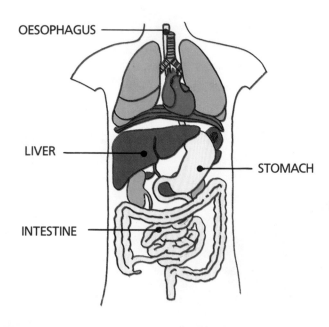

OESOPHAGUS

LIVER

STOMACH

INTESTINE

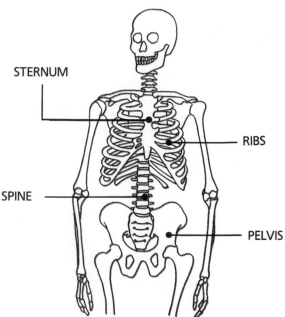

STERNUM

RIBS

SPINE

PELVIS

The Respiratory System

When we breathe in, a process we call inspiration, air first passes to the back of the mouth and nose (throat and pharynx) where it is warmed and moistened. The pharynx forms a short common pathway of air and food and ends by dividing into two tubes – oesophagus (gullet) and trachea (windpipe). The oesophagus lies behind the trachea in the neck and takes food and drink to the stomach. Air enters the trachea through the larynx (voice box), which can be felt in the front of the upper neck as the Adam's Apple and contains the vocal cords which produce the voice. Food is normally prevented from entering the larynx by a valvelike flap called the epiglottis. During swallowing the epiglottis closes off the larynx, but during breathing it opens to allow air through. Normally it is impossible to breathe and swallow at the same time, but in the unconscious or semi-conscious casualty this protection may be lost. That is why such a casualty should not be given anything to eat or drink. If solids or liquid pass into the larynx and trachea they obstruct the passage of air into the lungs. In addition, inhaled food or vomit is highly irritant and may cause severe or even fatal pneumonia.

The trachea ends in the upper part of the chest by dividing into two main tubes (the bronchi), one to each lung. These continue to divide into smaller and smaller bronchi until they end in very small thin-walled air sacs known as alveoli, each one of which is only a fraction of a millimetre across. Altogether there are about 300 million alveoli in the lungs and if they were all opened out and laid flat they would cover an area nearly as large as a tennis court. Around the alveoli and in close contact with them are equally thin walled blood vessels known as capillaries. Although the air and blood never mix, they are so close that oxygen (O_2) is able to pass from the alveoli into the blood. At the same time another gas, carbon dioxide (CO_2), passes from the blood into the alveoli. Carbon dioxide is a waste product (which is formed when oxygen is used up to produce energy) and it is got rid of as we breathe out.

The respiratory passages are lined by cells covered with cilia (tiny hairs), and kept moist by glands which produce a sticky material known as mucus. Dust, germs and other particles are caught on these cilia and may be coughed up together with the mucus as sputum (phlegm).

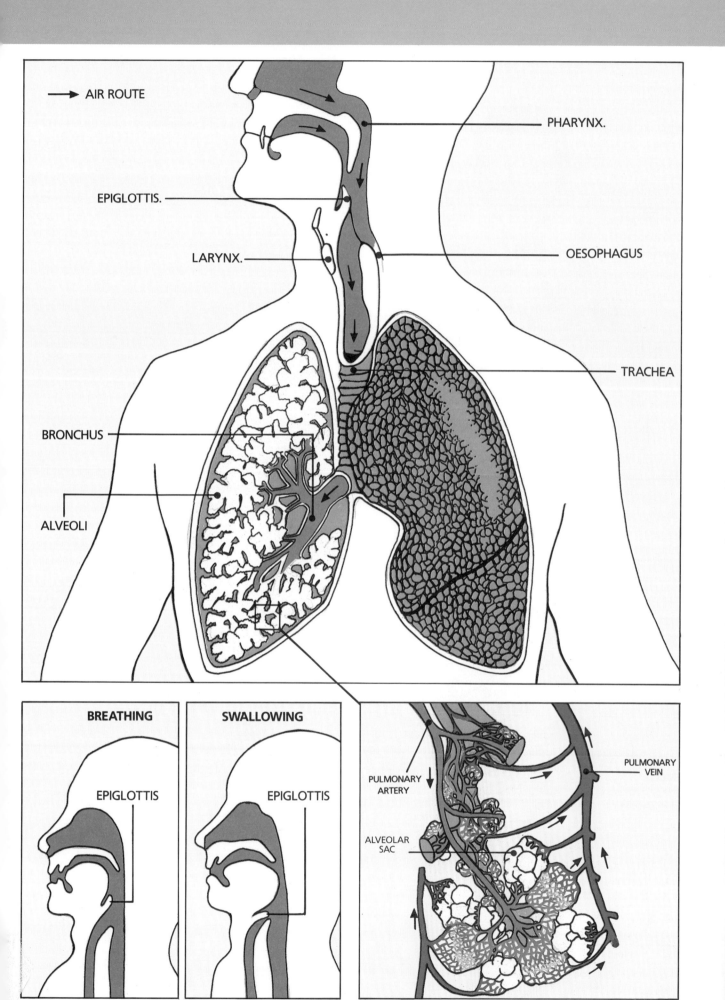

AIR ROUTE

PHARYNX.

EPIGLOTTIS.

OESOPHAGUS

LARYNX.

TRACHEA

BRONCHUS

ALVEOLI

BREATHING

SWALLOWING

EPIGLOTTIS

EPIGLOTTIS

PULMONARY
ARTERY

PULMONARY
VEIN

ALVEOLAR
SAC

Breathing

BREATHING-IN /INSPIRATION

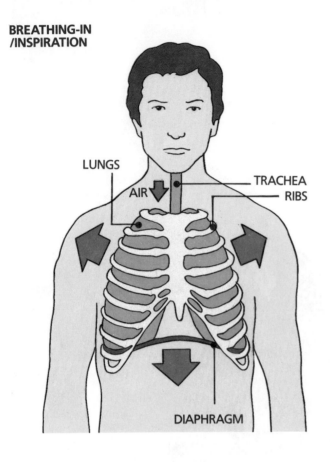

LUNGS

AIR

TRACHEA

RIBS

DIAPHRAGM

BREATHING-OUT/ EXPIRATION

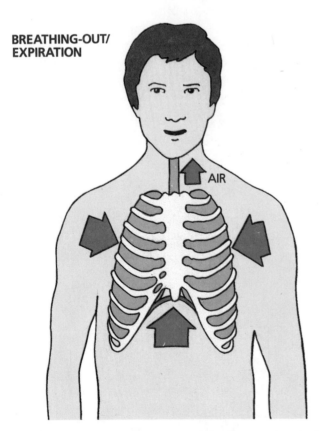

AIR

Lungs

The two lungs are cone-shaped and lie in the thorax (chest). They contain a great deal of elastic tissue so that when they are not full of air they tend to collapse down to a smaller size. They are protected by the sternum (breast bone) in front, the spine (vertebral column) behind, and the ribs which curve downwards and forwards from the spine. Between the ribs are muscles (intercostal muscles) which help in the action of breathing. The chest is closed below and separated from the abdomen by the diaphragm, which is a dome-shaped sheet of muscle attached to the spine and the lower ribs. Thus the whole thoracic cage is a closed and airtight box which contains the lungs, heart and major blood vessels.

Breathing

During inspiration the diaphragm contracts, so that its dome flattens. This increases the volume of the thoracic cavity and air is drawn into the lungs. When the diaphragm relaxes it returns to its domed shape and air is driven out of the lungs. At rest an adult normally breathes about 10 to 12 times a minute and a young child at about twice this speed. During exercise the rate increases and the diaphragm contracts more vigorously. In addition, each rib moves up and out rather like the movement of a bucket handle. This results in greater enlargement of the thoracic cavity and more air is drawn in. During hard exercise the volume of the thorax is increased still further by the lifting and pulling action of muscles in the neck and abdomen. These can readily be seen if you take a few very deep breaths whilst in front of a mirror.

Control of Breathing

Respiration is normally an involuntary act of which we are unaware. It is controlled by the Respiratory Centre which lies in the lower part of the brain. The various physical and chemical processes which go on inside the body use up oxygen and produce carbon dioxide. The Respiratory Centre is sensitive to the level of these two gases in the blood. During exercise the level of oxygen is reduced and the level of carbon dioxide goes up. The Respiratory Centre is particularly sensitive to the rise in carbon dioxide and sends messages through nerves to the muscles of respiration so that the rate and depth of breathing is increased. This results in more oxygen entering the blood and more carbon dioxide being removed. Deliberate overbreathing (hyperventilation) hardly increases the amount of oxygen in the blood as it is already nearly saturated, but it reduces the carbon dioxide level. This can produce dizziness or even loss of consciousness.

Blood Circulation

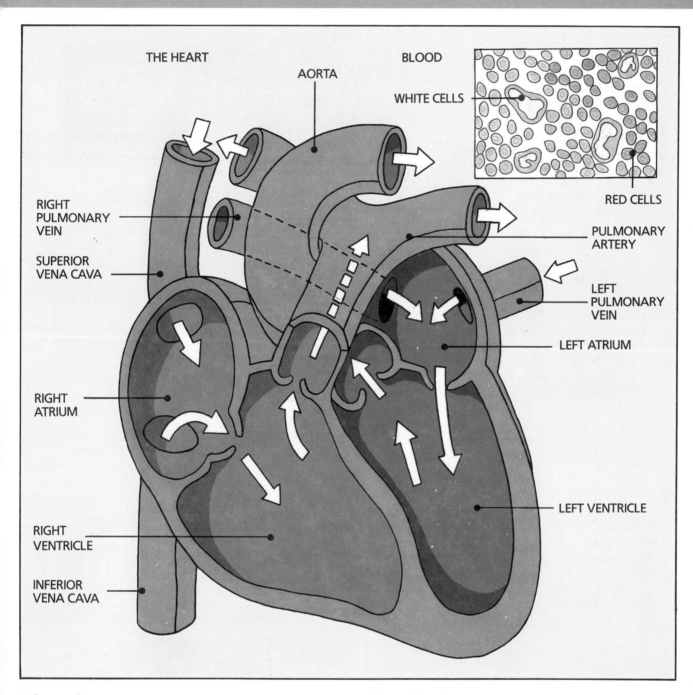

THE HEART

AORTA

BLOOD

WHITE CELLS

RED CELLS

RIGHT PULMONARY VEIN

SUPERIOR VENA CAVA

PULMONARY ARTERY

LEFT PULMONARY VEIN

LEFT ATRIUM

RIGHT ATRIUM

LEFT VENTRICLE

RIGHT VENTRICLE

INFERIOR VENA CAVA

Blood

The main function of the blood is to circulate oxygen, carbon dioxide, digested and absorbed food, water and other substances round the body; it also helps in the body's defence against infection and it plays an important part in maintaining a constant body temperature.

Blood is made up of about 55 per cent fluid (plasma) and 45 per cent cells. Dissolved in the plasma are many different substances including sugar and other forms of food. The cellular part consists mostly of red blood cells (red corpuscles) of which there are about 5 million in a drop the size of a pin head. When blood has taken up all the oxygen it can, it becomes bright red in colour but it becomes a darker blue-red when it loses its oxygen to the tissues. Blood also contains white cells whose main function is to fight infection. The smallest particles to be found are the platelets, which help in the process of blood clotting.

Circulation

The circulatory system consists of three parts: the blood, the heart, and the blood vessels (arteries, capillaries and veins).

The heart is a hollow muscular organ a little larger than a man's fist. It lies in the lower part of the chest between the two lungs, with the sternum in front and the vertebral column behind. It extends somewhat to the left side so that the heartbeat can be felt a little below the left nipple. There are four chambers inside the heart; the two upper ones collect blood and are known as atria; the two lower ones are the main pumps, and are known as ventricles. The left ventricle is stronger than the right ventricle as it has to pump blood round the whole of the body, whereas the right ventricle has to pump blood only to the lungs. Although both sides of the heart are joined together and beat as one, blood cannot pass directly from one side to the other, but first has to travel through the lungs. At rest, the heart beats about 72 times a minute.

Blood Circulation

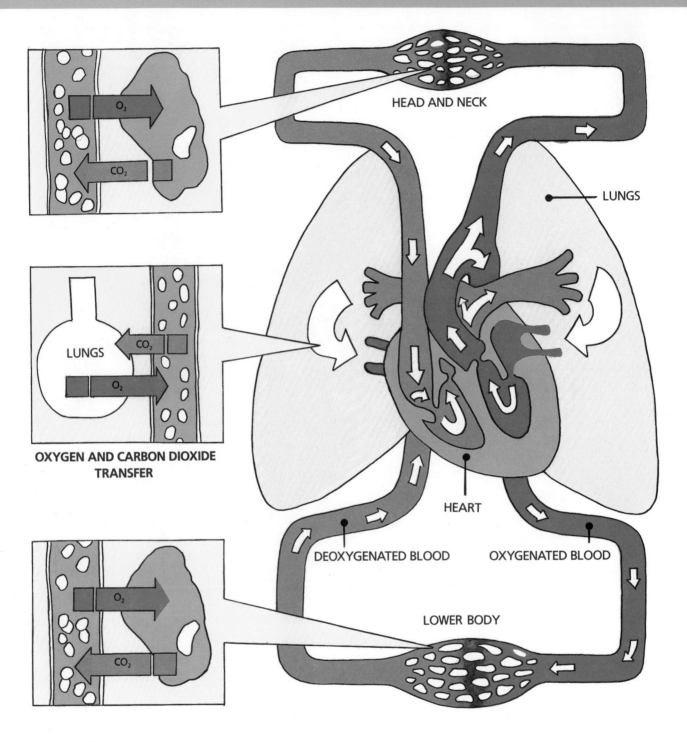

HEAD AND NECK

LUNGS

OXYGEN AND CARBON DIOXIDE
TRANSFER

HEART

DEOXYGENATED BLOOD

OXYGENATED BLOOD

LOWER BODY

After returning from its journey round the body, blood enters the right atrium. This blood has given up much of its oxygen and is carrying carbon dioxide back to the lungs. From the right atrium it passes through a non-return valve to the right ventricle. When the heart contracts (beats) blood is forced out of the right ventricle through another non-return valve into the pulmonary artery. From there it is distributed to both lungs, passing through smaller and smaller blood vessels, until it reaches the capillaries which are in contact with the alveoli. These capillaries are so small that red blood cells find it a tight fit to pass along even in single file. After getting rid of carbon dioxide and picking up more oxygen, the blood returns from the lungs in one of four pulmonary veins, two from each lung. This blood contains a high level of oxygen. After entering the left atrium it passes into the left ventricle, again through

a non-return valve. From the left ventricle it is pumped through a final valve into the main artery of the body, the aorta.

The arteries carry blood away from the heart and divide into smaller and smaller branches until finally they end up as millions of capillaries which distribute blood to all the body tissues. Oxygen passes out of the blood into the body cells and carbon dioxide passes from the cells into the blood. This is now collected into progressively larger blood vessels known as veins, which take blood back to the heart. Finally, two main veins, the superior and inferior venae cavae, return blood to the right atrium and the process begins again. Blood flows continuously round and round in this way making more than a thousand circuits every 24 hours.

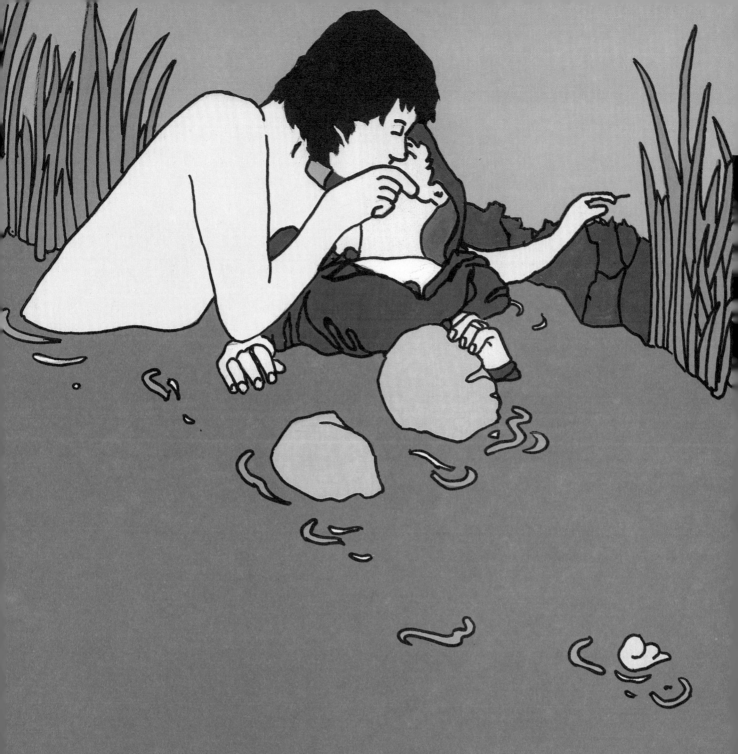

Chapter 3
Techniques of Resuscitation

Techniques of Resuscitation

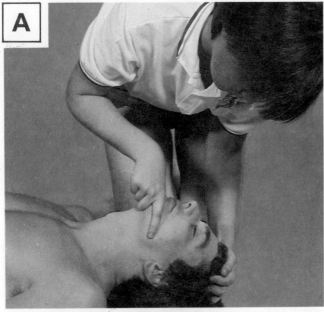

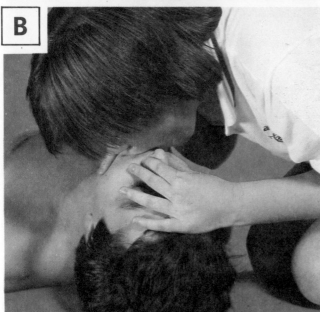

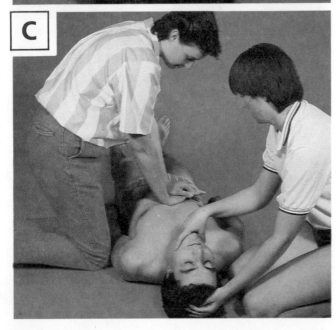

Resuscitation

Resuscitation is the act of reviving a nearly-dead or apparently dead person. It is necessary if breathing is inadequate (asphyxia) or the heart has stopped beating (cardiac arrest).

Asphyxia

This is the term used to describe any condition in which insufficient oxygen is reaching the tissues of the body to allow them to function normally. It may be due to:

a. Air being unable to reach the lungs (suffocation), e.g. tongue falling back and blocking the throat in an unconscious casualty; a foreign body stuck in the throat; strangulation; a child's head in a plastic bag.

b. Inadequate breathing movements, e.g. injury to the chest or muscles of respiration; deep unconsciousness; drug overdose; electric shock.

c. Failure of the blood to carry oxygen, e.g. carbon monoxide poisoning; loss of blood from bleeding.

d. Drowning: There is a mixture of factors, e.g. suffocation due to inhaled water in the air passages; interference with the transfer of oxygen from the lungs to the blood due to fluid secreted in to the alveoli (see Chapter 5).

Cardiac Arrest

This is the term used to indicate that the heart is no longer pumping blood round the body. The heart may stop beating either because its muscle is not contracting at all (asystole) or because it is twitching in a completely irregular and ineffective way (ventricular fibrillation). In neither case is there any circulation of blood or a pulse to be felt. The difference is important only when a doctor or paramedical person is available to apply specialised corrective treatment, and in any case cannot be diagnosed without an electrocardiogram (ECG). The techniques of resuscitation are the same whichever form cardiac arrest takes.

Cardiac arrest may be due to:

a. Direct damage to the heart muscle: heart attack (coronary thrombosis); electric shock.

b. Failure of the heart due to lack of oxygen: any of the causes of asphyxia (see above).

If a casualty stops breathing or suffers a cardiac arrest, it is only a short time before he dies from lack of oxygen. The brain is the most sensitive part of the body; within seconds of the heart stopping consciousness will be lost, and within a few minutes death will occur. Resuscitation must be started as soon as possible. The stages are:

● Ensuring an adequate airway
● Artificial ventilation by the Expired Air method
● Restoration of the circulation by External Chest Compression

As an aid to memory this can be thought of as:

A = Airway
B = Breathing
C = Circulation

Expired Air Resuscitation

Expired Air Resuscitation (EAR), sometimes known as the "kiss of life," has been shown to be much more effective than any other technique of artificial ventilation that does not rely on special equipment. Basically, it consists of the rescuer blowing air into a casualty's lungs by applying his own mouth to the casualty's mouth or nose. Although the air which the rescuer breathes out only contains 16 per cent oxygen compared with 21 per cent in the atmosphere, this is quite enough to keep the casualty alive.

Even if the casualty is in fact still breathing, EAR is harmless. Indeed, if respirations are weak they can be greatly helped by EAR applied at the same time.

The method can be taught easily to all age groups but its one main drawback is that it can be unpleasant for the rescuer. Casualties, particularly from drowning, often vomit and this may necessitate a change from mouth-to-mouth to mouth-to-nose resuscitation. The two methods have been shown to be equally effective in achieving ventilation.

External Chest Compression

External Chest Compression (ECC) will maintain circulation of the blood when the heart has stopped, and it may stimulate it into beating again. It consists of rhythmical compressions of the casualty's chest, achieved by the rescuer pressing down with his hands on the sternum (breast bone). There is some risk of damage to the heart, chest wall and abdominal organs during ECC. This risk is far outweighed by its lifesaving potential, but it does mean that it is vital to be sure of the diagnosis of cardiac arrest before starting.

It is important to remember that ECC and EAR, even when applied skilfully, may not result in the casualty's recovery if too much damage has occurred to the heart or there has been a delay before resuscitation has been started. Provided the rescuer has applied the techniques in a correct and careful manner he should have no cause for self-criticism whatever the outcome.

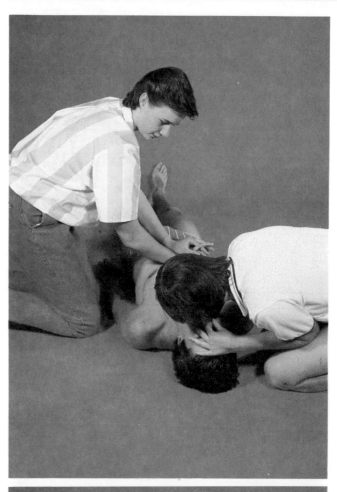

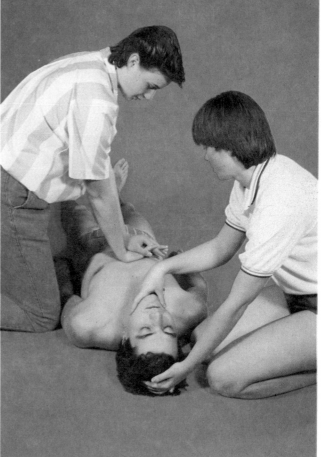

Sequence of Resuscitation

1 Check whether casualty is conscious.

2 Check whether casualty is breathing.

3 If unconscious and not breathing: turn him on his back.

4 Obtain a clear airway.

5 Start EAR if necessary.

6 Check casualty's pulse.

7 Start ECC if necessary.

8 Combine EAR and ECC (with an assistant if available).

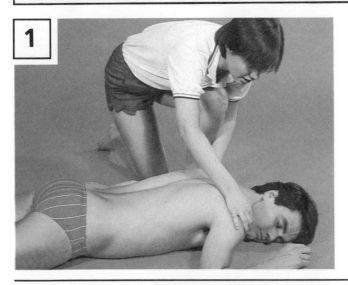

1. Check Whether Casualty is Conscious

Gently shake his shoulders and say loudly "Are you awake? Can you hear me?"

● If he responds by answering or moving, check that his breathing is normal (see below). If so, leave him in the position in which you find him (provided he is not in further danger) and check for any injury before trying to move him.

● If he is unconscious or you are not sure that his breathing is normal......

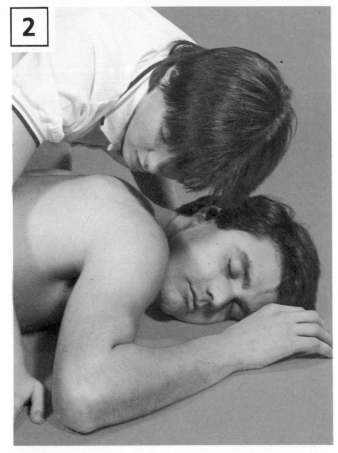

2. Check Whether Casualty is Breathing

Look for movement of the chest.

Feel and listen at the mouth for breathing, which should be quiet – a wheeze or rattle indicates obstruction.

Look for cyanosis – this is a bluish discolouration of the face, ears and nails which shows that the blood contains very little oxygen.

● If he is breathing quietly, place him in the Recovery Position (see page 26) unless this would aggravate an injury.

● Keep him under close observation and keep checking that he is breathing freely.

● If he is not breathing, if breathing is obstructed or if in any doubt......

3. Turn Casualty Onto His Back

Kneel by his side and place the arm nearer to you above his head.

Turn his head to face away from you.

Grasp his far shoulder with one hand and his hip with the other, at the same time clamping his wrist to his hip.

With a steady pull roll him over against your thighs.

Lower him gently to the ground on his back, supporting his head and shoulders as you do so; place his extended arm by his side.

It is important to turn the casualty over as quickly as possible whilst exercising great care, particularly not to injure his head.

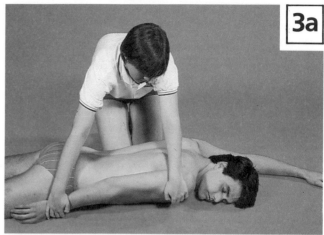

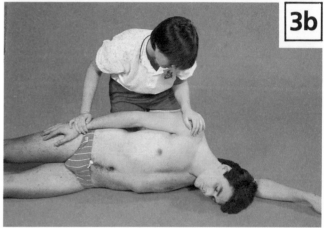

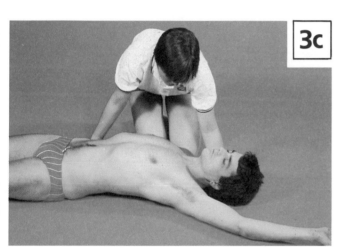

4. Obtain a Clear Airway

With the casualty on his back, quickly remove any debris or **loose** false teeth from his mouth – leave well-fitting dentures in place.

Loosen tight clothing around his neck.

Lift his chin with the fingers of one hand placed under the bony part of the jaw, near the point of the chin.

At the same time extend his neck by pressing downwards, just above his forehead, with your other hand; this will often allow breathing to restart, or obstructed breathing to improve.

● If breathing does not become normal......

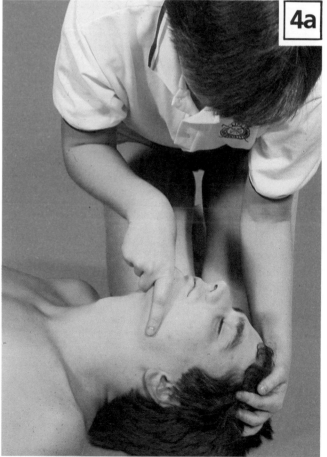

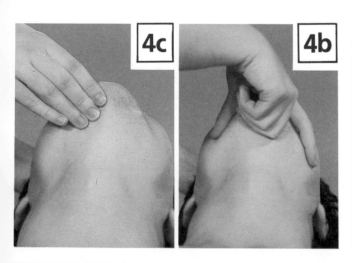

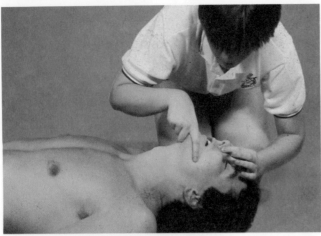

5. Start Expired Air Resuscitation

Maintain chin lift and neck extension.

Pinch the soft part of his nose closed with finger and thumb.

Allow the casualty's mouth to open a little, but maintain chin lift.

Take a full deep breath and place your lips around his mouth, making sure you have a good seal.

Breathe steadily into his mouth, watching from the corner of your eye for his chest to rise.

Maintaining chin lift and neck extension, take your mouth away from the casualty, take another full breath and repeat the sequence as above.

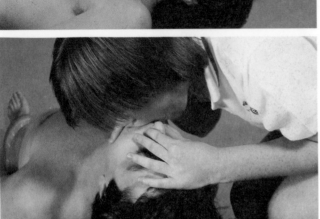

Notes:

a. Only a small amount of resistance to breathing should be felt, and each inflation should take between one-and-a-half and two seconds.

b. If you try and inflate too quickly resistance will be greater and less air will get into the lungs.

c. You should aim to breathe out to a comfortable point, NOT to empty your own lungs completely.

d. The two initial breaths should be completed in 5 to 8 seconds.

● If breathing does not restart during or immediately after the two initial breaths of EAR......

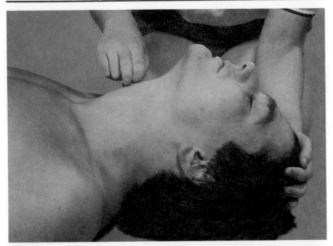

6. Check Casualty's Pulse

The best pulse to feel in an emergency is the carotid, which is found in the neck.

Ensure that the casualty's neck is extended.

Feel for the "Adams Apple" – a hard piece of cartilage in the midline of the neck about halfway between chin and upper part of the sternum. It is more prominent in men.

Slide two fingers from the "Adams Apple" sideways until they meet a strap-like muscle. Just beneath this can be felt the pulse.

Feel for five seconds before deciding it is absent.

● If the pulse is present:

Maintain chin lift and neck extension.

Repeat breaths of EAR at a rate of one every five seconds, taking about one-and-a-half to two seconds to inflate the casualty's chest.

Watch for the chest to rise and then fall, showing that the inflations are effective.

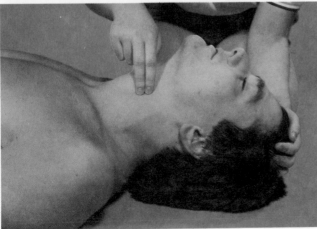

● **If the pulse is absent:** assume that cardiac arrest has occurred provided the casualty is:

- Still unconscious

- Making no movement or shivering

- "Deathly" pale or blue

7. Start External Chest Compression

Ensure that the casualty is on a flat, firm surface.

Feel for the lower borders of the rib cage, removing outer clothing if necessary. Identify the lower end of the sternum, which is where the two rib borders meet. Find the notch at the top of the sternum.

From these two landmarks locate the centre of the sternum.

Place the heel of one hand on the centre of the lower half of the sternum, with your other hand on top. Keep your arms straight and your fingers interlocked and raised to ensure that pressure is not applied over the ribs.

With your arms straight, press down vertically on the sternum.

Release the pressure, then repeat at a rate of about one compression a second (60-80 per minute).

Notes:

a. In an unconscious adult you should aim to press down approximately 4-5 centimetres and apply only enough pressure to achieve this.

b. At all times the pressure should be firm, controlled and applied vertically. Erratic or violent action is dangerous.

c. Try and spend about the same time in the compressed as the released phase.

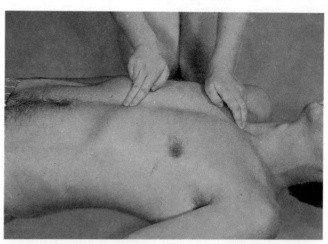

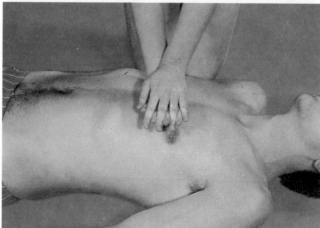

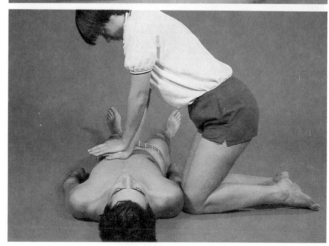

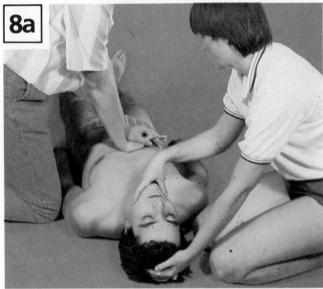

8a

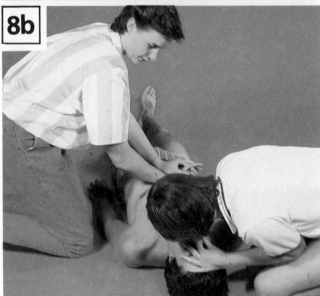

8b

8. Combine External Chest Compression with Expired Air Resuscitation (CPR)

It is essential to combine EAR with ECC in order that the blood which is being artificially circulated should contain adequate amounts of oxygen.

● If you are on your own:

After 15 compressions of ECC immediately lift the chin and extend the neck.

Give two full breaths of EAR.

Return immediately to ECC without waiting for expiration to occur.

Continue resuscitation by alternating 15 compressions with 2 inflations.

● With an assistant practised in Resuscitation:

Quickly decide who is to undertake EAR. This rescuer should:

Obtain a good airway with chin lift and neck extension.

Immediately after each fifth compression give a full breath of EAR.

Maintain jaw lift and neck extension as ECC is resumed, at a rate of about one per second, without waiting for expiration to occur.

Repeat a full breath between each fifth and sixth compression, interrupting the regular cycle of ECC just long enough to allow inflation to take place.

● With an untrained assistant:

Continue to give combined ECC and EAR yourself in a ratio of 15:2, whilst instructing him and demonstrating the technique.

Allow him to take over either ECC or EAR after you have completed two inflations of EAR.

Change to a ratio of five compressions to one inflation.

● Continue Resuscitation

If during combined ECC and EAR the casualty makes a movement or takes a spontaneous breath, check the carotid pulse to see if the heart is beating. Otherwise only interrupt resuscitation after about one minute and then at intervals of approximately three minutes. Take no more than five seconds to confirm that no pulse is present.

If breathing restarts but remains very shallow, or if cyanosis is still present, EAR should be continued. Breaths should then be given at the same time and rate as the spontaneous respiration in order to supplement these.

In the absence of obvious recovery of the casualty, resuscitation should continue:

a. Until medically qualified help arrives, or

b. The rescuer(s) become(s) totally exhausted.

Summary

Check whether casualty is conscious: Shake and call.

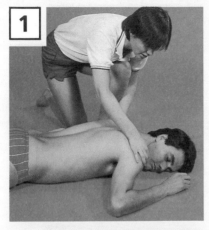

Check whether casualty is breathing: Look, feel and listen.

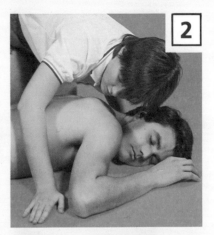

If unconscious and not breathing: Turn him on to his back.

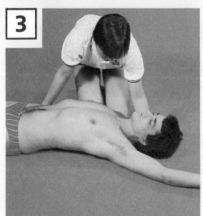

Obtain a clear airway: Check the mouth, lift the chin and extend the neck.

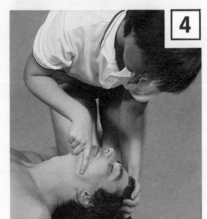

Start Expired Air Resuscitation: Give two inflations.

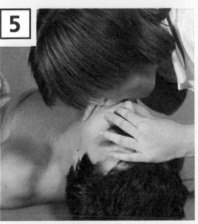

Check casualty's pulse: Feel for carotid pulse in neck. If pulse is present: Continue EAR – one inflation every five seconds.

If pulse is absent:

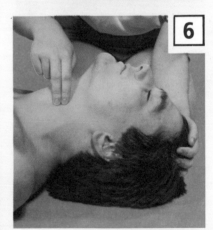

Start External Chest Compression: Hands placed on centre of lower half of sternum – compression rate 60-80 a minute.

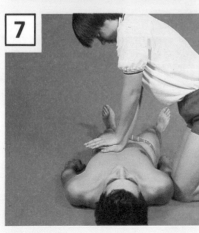

Combine EAR and ECC: One rescuer – 15 compressions to 2 inflations; Two rescuers – 5 compressions to 1 inflation.

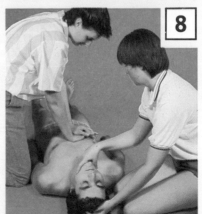

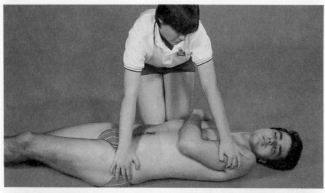

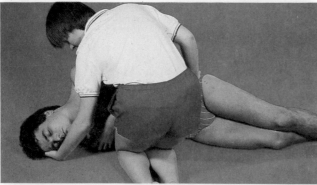

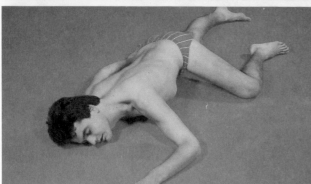

When heartbeat returns

When you are sure that a normal heartbeat has returned and the casualty is breathing on his own without any signs of obstruction you should:

Maintain a good airway and check at frequent intervals that the pulse and respiration remain normal.

Quickly examine the casualty for any injuries, in particular checking for bleeding.

Move him as little as possible, but ensure that he is sheltered from wind and rain, and is warm. Then......

Place Casualty in the Recovery Position

With the casualty on his back, kneel at his side and draw his far arm across his upper chest.

Tuck his nearer hand under his buttock.

Cross his far lower leg over the nearer one.

Take a firm grip of his far hip and shoulder and roll him carefully towards you. Support his head with your other hand to prevent injury.

Allow the weight of his body to rest against your thighs and lower his head carefully to the ground.

Place his upper arm and thigh at right angles to his body. This supports the weight of his chest and abdomen and keeps them clear of the ground, making it easier for him to breathe.

Adjust his lower arm so that it is behind and close to his body.

Keep his airway clear by tilting his head back, holding the jaw forward and mouth open.

Keep the casualty under close observation.

Be prepared to restart resuscitation if necessary.

● ALTERNATIVE METHOD

If the casualty is very heavy, it may be difficult to roll him towards you by gripping his shoulder and hip. In this case......

After tucking his nearer forearm under his buttock, bend his far leg by lifting behind the knee, and tuck that foot under his nearer knee.

Take a firm grip of the bent knee, and use your other hand to steady his head. Roll him carefully towards you.

Continue as above.

Observation

Whilst waiting for medical assistance to arrive all casualties should be observed carefully, especially in the early stages after resuscitation and when they are unconscious. Unless there is no-one else available to go and get help, you should remain with the casualty and watch for any signs of deterioration in his physical state. Continual reassurance can be very comforting and may help to reduce the risk of shock.

Problems during resuscitation

Difficulty with Inflation

If during EAR by the mouth-to-mouth technique, difficulty is experienced in inflating the casualty's chest:

Try to lift the chin further and increase neck extension.

Recheck that his mouth is clear of any loose obstruction.

Make sure that your lips are well sealed around his mouth.

If still in difficulty, change to the mouth-to-nose technique:

Release his nose and close his mouth.

Seal your mouth around his nose and breathe in steadily as for the mouth-to-mouth technique.

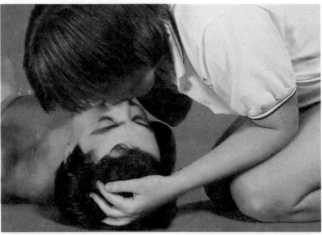

Vomiting

This commonly occurs during or immediately following successful resuscitation. The danger is that stomach contents will enter the air passages and lungs, not only interfering with respiration, but subsequently causing a particularly severe form of pneumonia. Immediate action is essential.

Turn the casualty away from you, keep him on his side and use your elbow and forearm to prevent him toppling on to his front.

Ensure that his head is turned towards the floor and his mouth is at the lowest point, thus allowing vomit to drain away.

Clear any residual debris from his mouth with your fingers.

Immediately turn him on to his back, re-establish an airway, and continue EAR at the normal rate of one inflation every five seconds. (The preliminary two inflations are not required.)

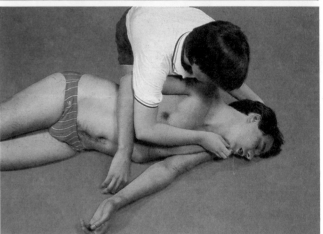

Air in Stomach

If neck extension and chin lift are not adequate enough to produce a clear airway, extra force is needed during EAR to blow air past the obstruction. This may drive air down the oesophagus (gullet) into the stomach. As the stomach distends, it interferes with the downward movement of the diaphragm and further reduces inflation of the lungs. There is also an increased risk that the casualty may vomit.

If distention of the stomach is seen (a swelling appearing in the abdomen below the left lower ribs) an attempt should be made to improve the casualty's airway. Chin lift and neck extension should be increased if possible.
No attempt should be made to apply pressure over the stomach as this is very likely to induce vomiting. Provided a clear airway is maintained the air in the stomach is likely gradually to escape.

Broken Ribs

During ECC one or more ribs may be heard to break. In elderly people, or those with particularly rigid chests, this may be unavoidable. It is far more likely to occur if the pressure used to compress the sternum is excessive, or if the hands are incorrectly placed on the sternum with pressure no longer being applied directly downwards towards the spine. If a rib does break, no action should or can be taken during resuscitation, which should continue uninterrupted. After recovery, the casualty may be expected to be in some pain.

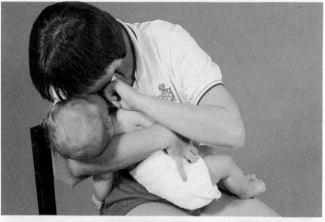

Resuscitation of Babies

When carrying out EAR, apply your mouth over the baby's mouth and nose. In spite of the small size of the baby's lungs the resistance to inflation is about that of an adult. The same effort therefore is needed during EAR, but the amount of air to fill the lungs is much less. Blow in fairly slowly, stopping as you see the chest rise. Increase the rate to 20-25 times a minute.

For ECC, the pressure of two fingers is enough. The compression rate should be about 100 per minute, and the depth of compression 1.5-2.5 centimetres.

For both EAR and ECC a baby may be held in your arms. Sufficient support for compression can be given by placing one hand underneath the baby's back.

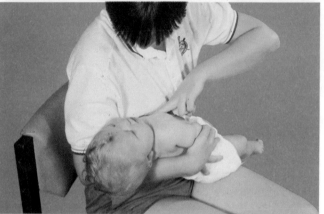

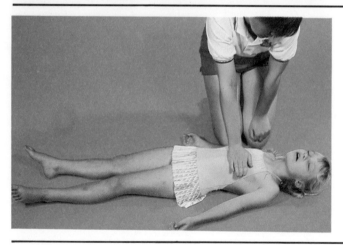

Resuscitation of Children

Whether mouth-to-mouth or mouth-to-mouth-and-nose is used for EAR depends upon the difference in size between you and the child. You will have to make a judgement about this and about the degree of pressure and rate of inflation required.

For children up to about the age of 10 years, ECC should be carried out using one hand only. The rate of compression will depend upon the age and size of the child, varying between about 100 compressions a minute for a baby and the usual adult rate of 60-80 compressions a minute for a 10-year-old child. The depth of compression should be 2.5-3.5 centimetres.

Tracheostomy

Very rarely, a Lifesaver may be faced with having to resuscitate a person who has undergone an operation for the removal of the voice box (laryngectomy). This will leave an opening to the windpipe in the front of the neck (tracheostomy). Expired Air Resuscitation should be carried out by the rescuer applying his mouth around the opening in the neck and inflating the lungs in the usual way.

Introduction

It is virtually impossible to carry out ECC in the water because of the difficulty in providing sufficient support behind the casualty's back. EAR is possible while swimming, but this requires a considerable degree of skill, a powerful swimming stroke and stamina. Every attempt should be made to find some form of support, such as the side of a boat or a floating aid. While performing EAR, the rescuer must endeavour to bring the casualty to shore as quickly as possible in order to carry out more effective resuscitation. To avoid delay the two initial breaths should be omitted. The mouth-to-nose technique is preferable in the water as this allows the free arm to hold on to support and to pass behind the casualty's neck to assist extension.

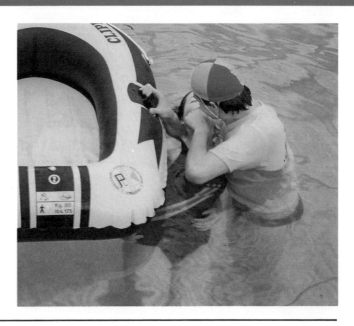

In Deep Water without Support

Support the casualty with one hand under the back of his head.

Quickly remove any debris or loose false teeth from his mouth.

Lift his chin and obtain good neck extension; use a cupped hand under his jaw so that no time is wasted changing grips before commencing the tow.

Carry out mouth-to-nose resuscitation but do not give the usual two initial inflations. Since you will need to tow the casualty to safety, and unsupported EAR is very tiring, give 1 inflation every 10 seconds, using the rest of the time to tow the casualty.

When giving an inflation, tread water with a strong leg kick. Keep the casualty's face out of the water and avoid twisting his neck.

Note:
This technique is very difficult to perform and should be attempted only by highly-trained lifesavers. In every case, high priority must be given to reaching support where resuscitation can be more effectively carried out.

Standing in Shallow Water

Support the casualty with one hand either under his far armpit or between his shoulder blades. Your forearm should pass under his neck to assist extension.

Quickly remove any debris or loose false teeth from his mouth.

Lift his chin in the usual way. The weight of his legs in the water will assist neck extension.

Ensure that water does not splash over the casualty's face.

Omit the usual two initial inflations. Carry out mouth-to-nose resuscitation at a rate of 1 inflation every 5 seconds, whilst walking with your casualty as quickly as possible to a point of safety.

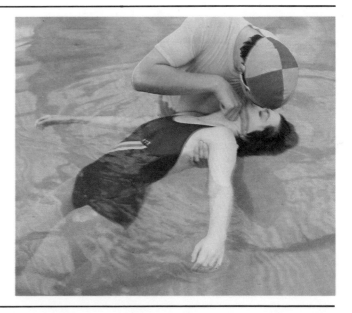

On Reaching Support

Support the casualty with your arm passing behind his neck to grip the bank or other means of support.

Use your other hand to obtain chin lift. There are two alternative methods by which this may be achieved. (See illustrations).

Unless breathing restarts . . .

● If you have not started EAR: quickly remove any debris or loose false teeth from the casualty's mouth and give two full inflations of EAR over 5–8 seconds.

● If you have already been giving EAR: give a further two inflations.

Then check for signs of cardiac arrest: Casualty still unconscious; making no movement; "deathly" pale or blue; no pulse felt.

● If you diagnose cardiac arrest, land the casualty as quickly as possible whether help is available or not.

● If his pulse is present, continue EAR for a further two or three inflations, or until you have recovered from the exertions of towing, then land the casualty, with assistance if available.

Once the casualty has been landed, resuscitation must be continued as long as necessary, and after-care instituted as detailed above.

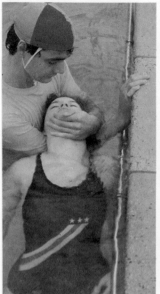 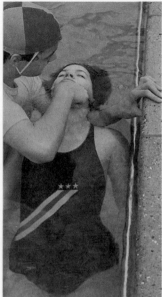

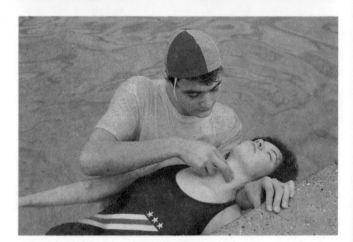

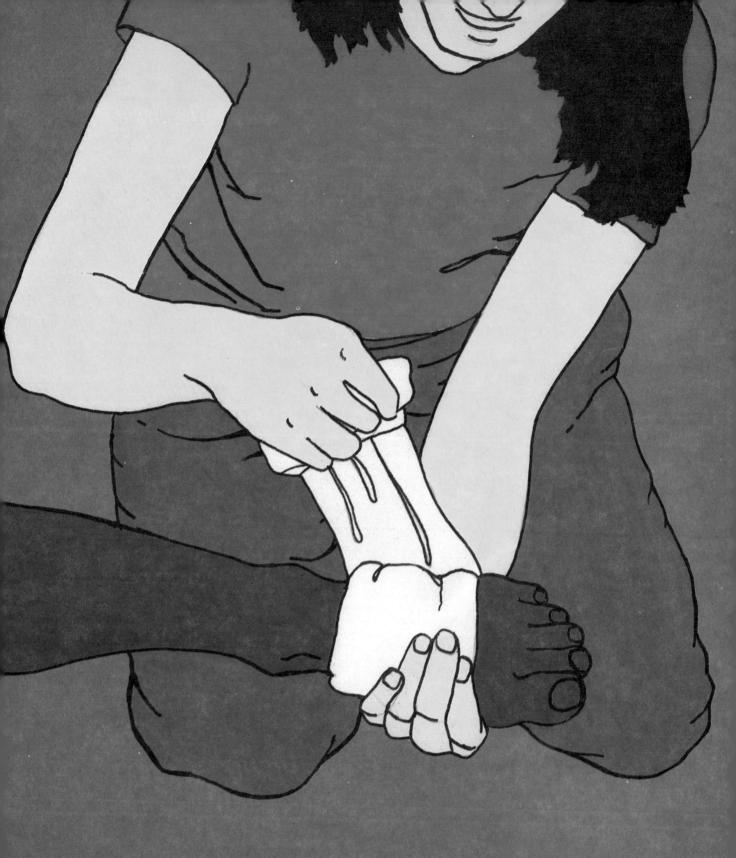

Chapter 4
General First Aid

First Aid

Diagnosis

Before it is possible to carry out First Aid, it is essential to know from what illness or injury the casualty is suffering. This is the process of making a diagnosis and consists of four stages:

History

This is **how** the illness began or the accident occurred. A conscious casualty should be carefully questioned about the events leading up to the incident. Clearly if the casualty is unconscious, then these details can be obtained only from witnesses. Knowing for example that a casualty hit his head when falling, will direct attention to possible injury of that part of the body. Again, if an unconscious casualty has been seen to jerk his limbs and foam at the mouth, this suggests that the cause of the unconsciousness is an epileptic fit. Always ask the casualty or available friends or relatives if he is known to suffer from any particular disease, or to be on any medical treatment, as this again may give a clue to the cause of the present illness. He may be carrying a card or wearing a bracelet that gives details of a condition from which he suffers, e.g. diabetes.

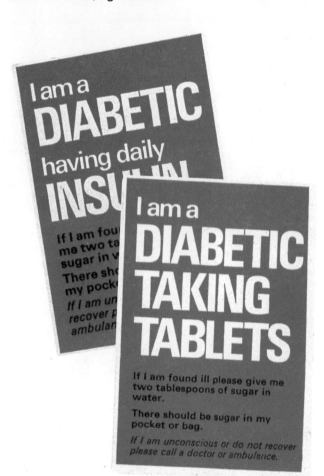

Symptoms

These are the ways in which the casualty tells you he **feels** unwell. He may volunteer that he is in pain, feels faint, sick etc. Always try and elicit as much detail as possible, such as the site of the pain, its nature, how long it has been present and whether he has had it before. After accidents, try and discover whether the casualty has any numbness or loss of muscle control since these symptoms may indicate damage to the nerve pathways, particularly injury to the spinal cord.

Signs

These are the abnormalities you **detect** in a casualty which indicate injury or disease. As soon as lifesaving and other urgent measures have been taken, it is important to make a quick but thorough examination of the whole of the casualty. This consists of listening, looking and feeling. **Listen** for abnormal breathing or choking, determine whether speech is normal and note whether the casualty is confused. **Look** at the casualty's general appearance, whether pale or cyanosed, sweaty, hot or cold, etc. Look also for any evidence of bleeding and for distorted limbs suggesting the presence of a fracture. **Feel** very gently for any areas of swelling or deformity of bones. Determine whether the casualty can move all four limbs.

Remember that to examine a casualty adequately, clothing may need to be removed. If necessary, do not hesitate to cut garments rather than risk further injury by trying to preserve them intact.

Records

It can be very helpful to subsequent medical attendants if a brief record can accompany the casualty to hospital. The points that should be noted are:

a. How the accident happened
b. How long the casualty has been unconscious
c. A record of his pulse rate and character (strong or weak; regular or irregular) taken every ten minutes
d. Injuries
e. An estimate of the amount of blood loss
f. Any treatment given
g. Times should be noted where possible and the rescuer should add his name and address

Minor Bleeding

The general principles of dealing with severe bleeding are given in Chapter 1. The same principles of treatment apply to minor cuts and grazes.

1. Apply direct pressure to the wound using your fingers or a pad of clean material if this is available. If the bleeding does not stop, do not disturb any dressings, but add more and bandage firmly.
2. If possible, raise the injured part above the level of the heart to reduce the flow of blood.
3. If the injury is anything other than very minor, take the casualty to a doctor or hospital.

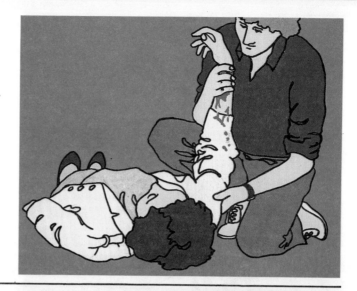

Choking

Choking occurs when a piece of food or other material is swallowed but goes down the trachea (windpipe) rather than the oesophagus (gullet). This results in blockage of the airway. If this blockage is only partial the casualty will usually be able to dislodge it by coughing, but if there is complete obstruction to the flow of air, this may not be possible. Unless help is given urgently the casualty will suffer from asphyxia, become unconscious and may die. Even a small piece of food such as peanut may cause serious obstruction because its presence can lead to muscle spasm in the region of the pharynx.

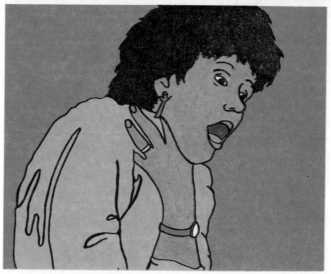

● **DIAGNOSIS**

a. The casualty may have been seen to be eating, or a child may have put an object into its mouth.
b. A casualty who is choking often grips his throat with his hand.
c. **With partial airway obstruction** the casualty will be distressed and coughing. Breathing may be noisy (wheezy).
d. **With complete airway obstruction** the casualty will be unable to speak, breathe or cough. Cyanosis will occur. His face may become congested with the veins in the neck standing out.

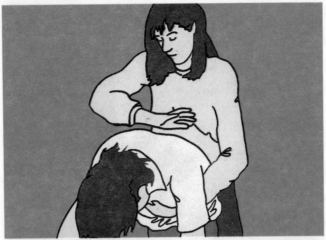

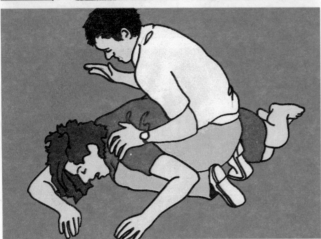

● TREATMENT

1. If the casualty is breathing, encourage him to continue coughing, but **do nothing else.**
2. If he shows signs of becoming weak or he stops breathing or coughing, leave the casualty in the position in which you find him, remove any obvious debris or loose false teeth from his mouth and carry out **back slapping.**

a. If he is standing or sitting
- Stand to the side and slightly behind him.
- Support his chest with one hand and lean him forwards.
- Give up to four sharp slaps between his shoulder blades with the heel of your other hand.

b. If he is lying
- Kneel beside him and roll him on to his side.
- Support his chest with your thigh.
- Give up to four sharp slaps as above.

The aim should be to relieve the obstruction with each slap rather than necessarily giving all four.

Note: It is important to distinguish between choking and a heart attack because the treatments are very different.

● HOW TO DISTINGUISH BETWEEN:

Choking	Heart Attack
Casualty often stands up and becomes agitated	Casualty usually sits down and becomes quiet
Casualty clutches neck	Casualty holds central chest
There is no pain	Casualty often complains of chest pain
Face is blue and congested	Face may be blue, but is often pale
Breathing may be absent or noisy	Breathing is usually rapid and quiet

Heart attack

Introduction

If one of the coronary arteries supplying blood to the heart suddenly becomes blocked, part of the heart muscle suffers injury. We call this a heart attack or coronary thrombosis. The damage may interfere with the pumping action of the heart, giving rise to heart failure and shock. Cardiac arrest can occur at any time. The most obvious symptom suffered by the casualty is chest pain.

● DIAGNOSIS

The casualty complains of:

a. A sudden, severe, crushing, tight or heavy pain in the centre of his chest which may spread to his arms, throat or back.

b. He often looks pale and sweaty and feels faint. There may be other signs of shock (see page 9).

c. Breathing may become difficult (see opposite page to distinguish the symptoms of a heart attack from those of choking).

● TREATMENT

1. Give the heart as little work to do as possible by placing the casualty in a half-sitting position.

2. Loosen tight clothing at the neck and waist.

3. Reassure him.

4. Check his breathing and pulse and be prepared to start CPR if necessary.

5. If he becomes unconscious but continues to breathe normally place him in the Recovery Position.

6. Obtain medical assistance urgently, preferably by calling an ambulance.

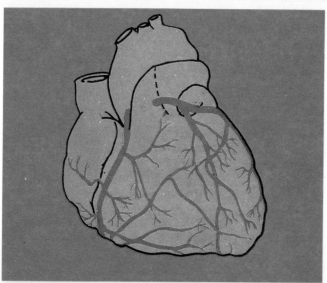

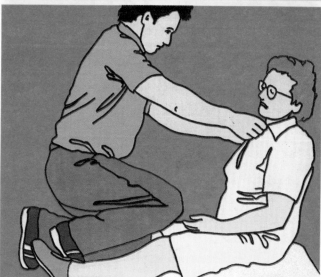

Fractures

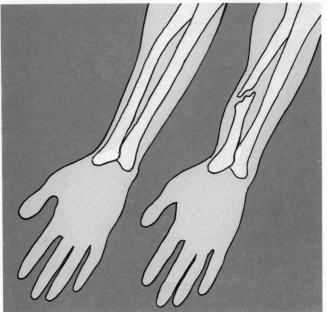

Introduction

A fracture is a break in a bone. It may be caused by a direct blow or an indirect force such as twisting. The sharp ends of the broken bone may damage other structures such as nerves, blood vessels and internal organs, or may penetrate the skin and allow infection to complicate the injury.

● DIAGNOSIS

a. The injury may have been witnessed and a cracking sound heard at the time.

b. Severe pain at the site of the injury is usual but not invariable.

c. Any movement of the affected part by the casualty is severely limited and makes the pain worse.

d. Swelling and deformity (irregularity) are often present where the injury occured. A limb may appear bent or irregular or be held in an unnatural position. Compare one side of the body with the other to recognise the differences.

● TREATMENT

1. Keep the casualty in the position in which he is found, unless he or you are in danger of further injury or exposure to the weather.

2. Cover any external wound with a clean dry cloth or dressing.

3. Move the broken part as little as possible. Support an upper limb by hand or in a sling if available. Immobilise a lower limb by the use of splints, or bandage the broken limb to the opposite one, putting pads under the bandages and between the legs to reduce pressure on the injured area.

4. Raise the supported limb to reduce pain and swelling.

5. Treat for shock.

6. Arrange to transport the casualty to hospital.

7. **Do not** move the injured part unnecessarily.

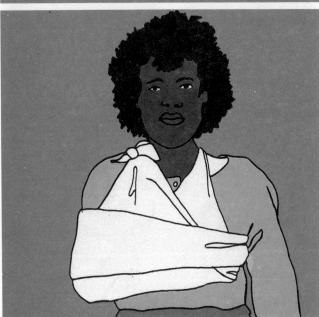

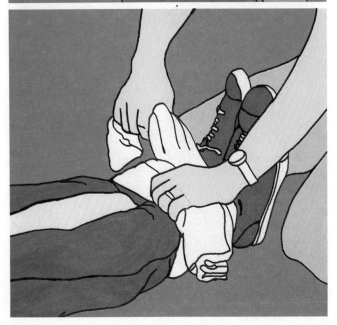

Burns

Introduction

Lifesavers may on occasion have to deal with burns resulting from flames, scalds, chemicals or electric currents. In each case the principles of management are the same.

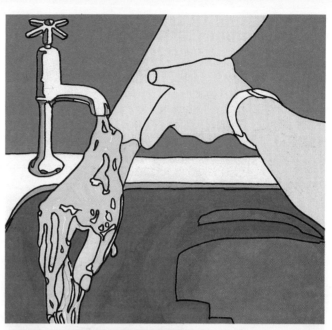

● DIAGNOSIS

a. Burns are usually obvious and the casualty will complain of severe pain. However, some serious burns may cause surprisingly little pain because the whole thickness of the skin, including the pain-sensitive nerves, is destroyed.

b. When a large area of the body has been burned, considerable quantities of fluid (plasma) may be lost, and this, together with the pain, may cause severe shock.

c. In an unconscious casualty always look for areas of scorching or reddening of the skin if a burn or scald is suspected.

● TREATMENT

1. The burnt area should be immersed in cold running water if possible and kept there for 10 minutes to draw heat out of the injured part.

2. If clothing or other material has become stuck to the burnt area **do not** attempt to remove this; it will have been sterilised by the heat and its removal will cause further damage.

3. Gently remove any rings, watches, straps etc. before the injured area starts to swell.

4. Cover the burn with a clean (preferably sterile) material and keep this in place with lightly applied bandages. **Do not** burst any blisters as this will let in infection.

5. Under no circumstances put any creams, oils, lotions, etc. on the affected parts.

6. Treat the casualty for shock if this is present.

7. Ensure that medical assistance is obtained according to the severity of the injury.

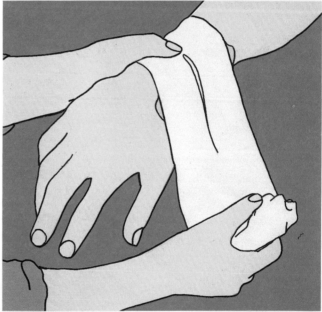

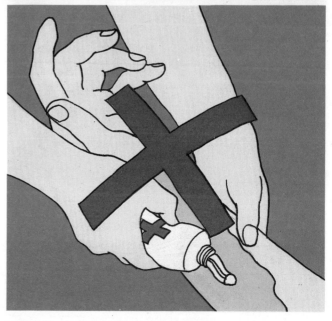

Electric Shock

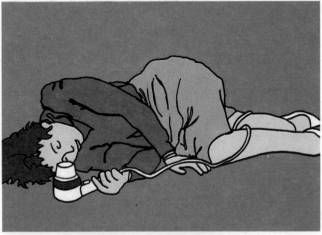

Introduction

Most accidents due to electricity occur from contact with the domestic supply. A few are due to lightning, and a few to contact with high voltage current such as that carried in power lines and overhead railway cables. The passage of the current through the body may produce the following effects:

a. Unconsciousness

b. Spasm of the muscles of respiration so that breathing stops; this is the commonest cause of death

c. Cardiac arrest due to ventricular fibrillation

d. Local burns at the points where the current entered and left the body. These burns are often deeper than they first appear.

● RESCUE

It is **essential** that the casualty is removed from contact with the electric supply before any attempt at rescue or resuscitation is made. This should be done as follows:

Domestic Voltage

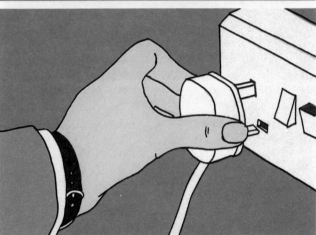

a. Switch off the current, remove the electric plug or wrench the cable free.

b. If this is not possible, stand on some dry material such as wood, a rubber mat or several layers of newspaper. Use a long piece of wood such as a broom handle or chair, or other dry non-conducting material such as rubber or folded newspaper to push the casualty out of contact with the electric source.

c. If this also is not possible, use a piece of rope or dry clothing to loop round the casualty's feet or arms to drag him away.

d. **At no time touch the casualty with bare hands until the current is disconnected.**

High Voltage

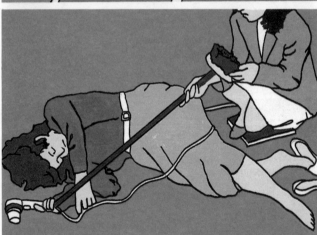

If a casualty is found in contact with, or within 20 metres of a high voltage current **keep well clear and make no attempt at rescue** until you are informed by the authorities that the power has been turned off. High-voltage electricity can arc considerable distances and any approach by the rescuer puts him in serious danger of electrocution as well.

● TREATMENT

1. If cardiac arrest has occured or breathing has stopped, carry out resuscitation immediately (see page 18).

2. If the casualty is unconscious but breathing normally, place him in the Recovery Position (see page 26).

3. Look for burns and treat them in the usual way (see page 37). If they are present, the casualty should receive medical attention as soon as possible as there may be considerable damage to deeper tissues even if the surface skin only appears mildly affected.

4. Carry out the appropriate actions for the prevention and treatment of shock. (see page 9).

5. If there is any suggestion that the casualty may have lost consciousness, or he appears "shaken," medical attention should be sought.

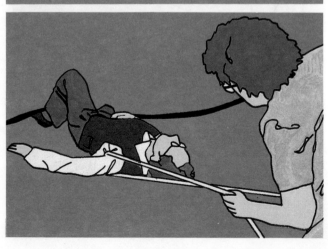

Gas and smoke inhalation

Introduction

In most cases of gas or smoke inhalation the problem is one of asphyxia because the casualty has been breathing air containing reduced concentrations of oxygen.

The commonest incident likely to be encountered is one involving carbon monoxide. This is an invisible, odourless gas which is found in the exhaust fumes from petrol engines. It is dangerous because it displaces oxygen already in the red blood cells, thereby producing asphyxia. Accidental or deliberate poisoning should be suspected if, for example, a car engine is heard behind closed garage doors.

Non-poisonous gases such as butane and propane may be found as cooking or lighting fuel in boats. They become dangerous if they escape in sufficient quantity to form a high proportion of the inspired air as this reduces the amount of oxygen available. Smoke has a similar effect, also causing coughing and choking.

● RESCUE

If the casualty is in a closed space and poisonous fumes are suspected **do not enter.** Call the Fire Brigade, stating the nature of the poisonous substance if known.

If carbon monoxide or a non-poisonous gas is suspected, doors and windows should be opened widely before entering the area.

Before going into a room filled with smoke, tie a dampened handkerchief over your mouth and nose. Then take a deep breath, go in, and try to pull the casualty out without having to breathe whilst inside.

If the casualty is behind a closed door which feels hot to the touch, or hot air is coming from under the door, **do not open it** as you may spread the flames and put yourself in danger. Call the Fire Brigade.

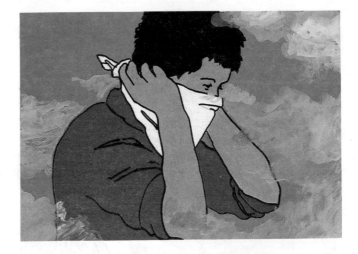

● TREATMENT

1. Do not attempt resuscitation whilst in a smoke or gas filled room.
2. If breathing has stopped, appears shallow, or is noisy, ensure that there is no obstruction or debris in the mouth. Extend the neck and lift the chin to establish a good airway. If breathing does not recommence, start Expired Air Resuscitation (see page 20). Make certain that you do not inhale the casualty's exhaled breath.
3. If the casualty is unconscious but breathing normally place him in the Recovery Position (see page 26).
4. Obtain urgent medical attention or call an ambulance.

Panic

Sometimes a casualty, but more commonly a bystander, may become so anxious about an emergency situation that he panics. This implies loss of normal emotional control and his behaviour may become irrational and even violent. If the person panicking is a friend or relative of someone involved in an incident, restraint may be needed to prevent him from putting himself in danger, for example by attempting rescue himself. Even a trained Lifesaver, if he shows signs of panic should be gently but firmly prevented from becoming involved in the rescue as his judgement will be clouded. Sometimes panic leads to hyperventilation (see page 14) and results in dizziness or loss of consciousness.

● TREATMENT
1. Reassure the sufferer.
2. Use as little restraint as necessary, but prevent him from becoming a danger to himself.
3. Do not slap him or return any physical violence.
4. Ensure that somebody stays with him until his manner and behaviour have returned to normal.

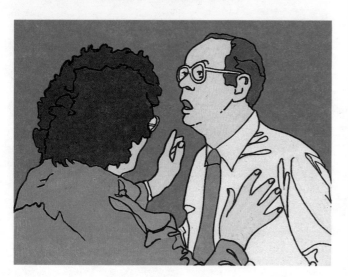

Handling and transporting the casualty

It is a general rule of First Aid that a casualty should be handled and moved as little as possible. This is particularly important if any injury to the spine is suspected (see page 44). Sometimes it is necessary to remove the casualty from further danger, or to move him in order to obtain further medical care. Considerable skill is required to lift casualties safely and comfortably, and it is the Society's policy to encourage all Lifesavers to take a First Aid course, such as that run by the St. John Ambulance, St. Andrew's Ambulance Association or the British Red Cross Society, where these techniques are taught.

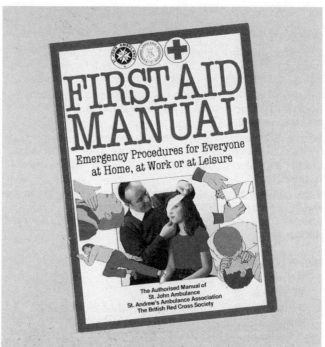

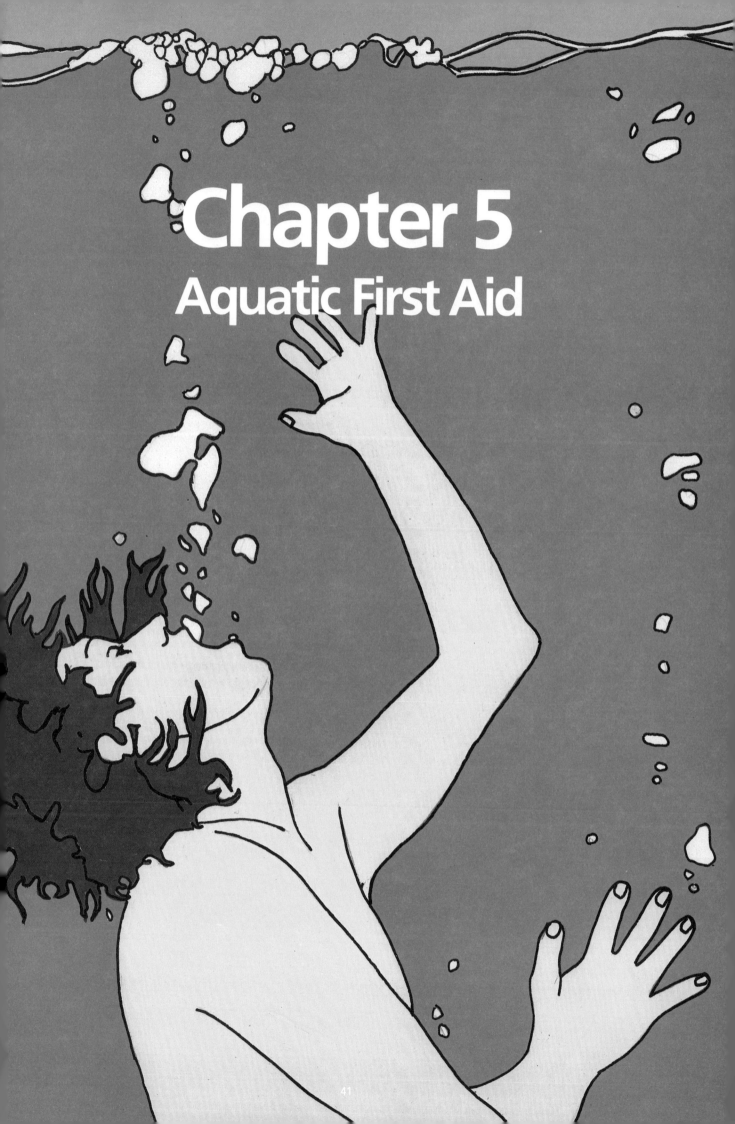

Chapter 5
Aquatic First Aid

Drowning

Introduction

Drowning is death caused by asphyxia (see page 18) following immersion in water; up to 800 people in the British Isles lose their lives this way each year. The term "near-drowning" is used if the casualty survives. Although the final cause of death is failure of air to get in to the lungs, there are often other factors which lead up to this and may therefore be considered causes of drowning. For example, a sudden debilitating illness, such as a stroke or heart attack, may result in the casualty falling into the water and being unable to help himself; the low sea temperatures around the British coast rapidly produce hypothermia (see Chapter 6) with consequent loss of muscle control and inhalation of water; in about 25% of fatal drowning incidents some degree of alcohol intoxication has been shown to be a contributory factor.

In most cases of drowning, relatively small quantities of water enter the lungs, but this is enough to interfere with the normal transfer of oxygen from the inspired air to the blood. The water also causes irritation, and results in an outpouring of fluid in to the alveoli which further impairs oxygen transfer. This "secondary drowning" can be delayed for up to 72 hours, so it is important to watch carefully any immersion victim even if he appears to have recovered fully.

There is little difference between the effects of inhaling small amounts of fresh or salt (sea) water. On the other hand, if the quantity reaching the lungs is large, fresh water leads to more rapid drowning because it is absorbed in to the blood stream and damages the red cells.

In about 10 per cent of cases of drowning (so called "dry drowning") water does not reach the lungs because of muscle spasm in the region of the larynx. This spasm also cuts off the air supply and produces asphyxia as in "wet" drowning.

During prolonged immersion, the water has a "squeezing" effect on the body causing loss of fluid (including blood plasma) through the kidneys. When the casualty is rescued, his body re-expands but there is now insufficient blood and fluid to fill the restored volume. As a result, blood circulation is inadequate and signs of shock may appear (see page 9). This condition is known as "post-immersion collapse" and was commonly seen after sea rescues during the Second World War.

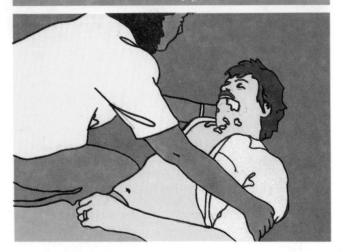

● TREATMENT

1. The priority of First Aid treatment is Cardiopulmonary Resuscitation.

2. If possible keep the casualty horizontal during rescue to counteract shock due to post-immersion collapse.

3. Do not waste time trying to drain water from the lungs; little is likely to be there and its removal is impossible.

4. Turn the casualty on to his back, clear obvious debris, seaweed etc. from the mouth, and if necessary start EAR. Continue with combined EAR and ECC (CPR) as required (see Chapter 3).

5. Drowning casualties often vomit or have froth around their mouths. This makes CPR unpleasant and the Lifesaver must be prepared to continue resuscitation under these conditions.

6. Do not stop CPR even in apparently hopeless cases; complete recovery has been reported after prolonged resuscitation even when the casualty has initially appeared dead.

7. Keep the casualty lying flat with his feet raised to prevent the effects of shock (see page 9).

8. All near-drowned casualties, those who have been successfully resuscitated, and any in whom aspiration of water is even suspected must be taken to hospital, however complete their apparent recovery, because of the risk of "secondary drowning."

Sub-aqua diving

Introduction

Skin and scuba diving are specialised pursuits which should be undertaken only by properly trained swimmers under the supervision of recognised sub-aqua clubs.

At ten metres (33 feet) depth of water, pressure on the body is double that at the surface; at twenty metres (66 feet) it is three times and at thirty metres (99 feet) it is four times surface pressure. This increased pressure can cause problems both during the dive and on returning to the surface.

Pressure during descent can rupture the eardrums causing pain and severe dizziness. Bleeding may occur both into the ears and into the sinuses, which are hollow spaces lying within the bones of the face and forehead; pain is the main symptom. Bleeding may also occur into the skin which can be unsightly, but is rarely serious.

As pressure increases, so any gas within the body becomes compressed and takes up less space. If a full breath is taken from scuba equipment whilst at depth and held during ascent to the surface, the gas expands and can cause rupture of the lungs. Air then escapes into the chest cavity (pneumothorax) and causes the lung to collapse, producing chest pain and difficulty in breathing. Air may also be forced into the blood stream, interfering with the circulation and resulting in unconsciousness, fits, dizziness, weakness or paralysis of limbs.

Decompression sickness (The Bends) can occur during or shortly after surfacing from a dive. Because of the increased pressure at depth any air breathed is at higher than surface pressure. Nitrogen (a gas forming nearly 80 per cent of air) is absorbed into the blood in large amounts. On surfacing rapidly, this nitrogen can no longer remain dissolved in the blood and forms bubbles. These give rise to pain in the joints and limbs, dizziness, confusion, impaired vision and vomiting. Permanent physical disability can result if correct and urgent treatment is not given.

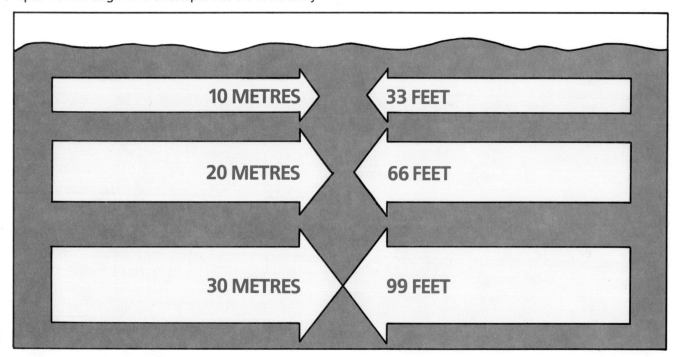

10 METRES	33 FEET
20 METRES	66 FEET
30 METRES	99 FEET

● DIAGNOSIS

Lifesavers should not waste time trying to make an exact diagnosis. The British Sub-Aqua Club discourages solo sport diving, so information about the incident can usually be obtained from the diver's partner. Treat as potentially serious any of the following which occur during or after diving:

a. Pain, particularly in the joints, ears and face which is not explained by visible external injury.

b. Abnormal behaviour, confusion or any interference with consciousness.

c. Any complaint of weakness, dizziness, nausea or impaired vision.

d. Bleeding from the ears or nose, or spontaneous bruising.

● TREATMENT

1. If cardiac arrest has occured or breathing has stopped, carry out resuscitation immediately (see Chapter 3).

2. In all other circumstances, the casualty's condition should still be considered potentially serious. Little can be done on the spot by the rescuer, other than reassuring the casualty and making him as comfortable as possible, preferably laying him down with his head and chest (heart) as low as possible in relation to the rest of his body.

3. Urgent transport to medical care should be arranged and it should be stressed that a **diving emergency** has occured, as treatment in a recompression chamber may be required.

Cramp

Introduction

This is a sudden, involuntary, painful contraction of a muscle. It becomes dangerous if it occurs, whilst the casualty is in the water because it may impair normal swimming actions. It can be caused by:

- Cold conditions
- Sudden or unusual exercise
- A blow or injury to a muscle
- Excessive loss of salt as in severe sweating

● DIAGNOSIS

a. The casualty complains of pain in a muscle, often in the calf or front of the trunk.

b. The affected muscle feels tight and hard and the casualty cannot relax it.

● TREATMENT

1. Stretch the muscle by straightening the limb. If the calf muscle is affected, straighten the knee and push the casualty's toes upwards.

2. If the abdominal muscles are involved, encourage the casualty to stand straight and arch his back slightly.

3. Rub the affected muscle gently.

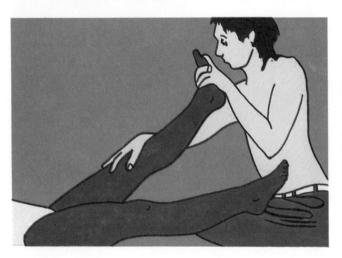

Spinal Injuries

Introduction

All spinal injuries are potentially serious because of the risk of damage to the spinal cord. This runs inside a tunnel made up of arches projecting from each of the vertebrae (blocks of bone) which make up the spine. Because of this protection most spinal injuries do not result in permanent disability. Diving accidents are, however, particularly hazardous as they produce a combination of vertical compression and forward flexion of the spine.

Damage to the Spinal cord is more serious if it occurs in the neck rather than in the back, because nerve pathways to both the upper and lower limbs are interrupted. A high neck injury may interfere with breathing and prove fatal. Damage to the spinal cord can give rise to paralysis of the arms and/or legs which may be partial, total, temporary or permanent.

In swimming pools spinal injuries may be associated with collisions at the foot of water slides (flumes) or with other swimmers or pool side or bottom. In open water, accidents usually occur when someone dives into shallow water and collides with the bottom. A swimmer picked up by a wave in surf conditions may be "dumped" on the bottom with consequent neck injury.

It is important to be aware that the spinal cord, unlike most other parts of the body, is unable to repair itself once damaged. Any paralysis that occurs therefore is usually permanent.

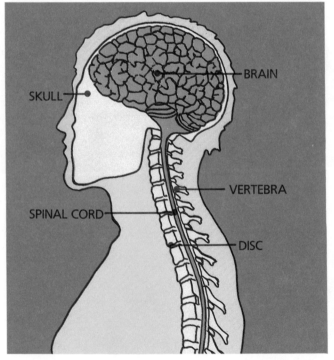

● DIAGNOSIS

a. The casualty may be seen to dive in to shallow water.

b. If paralysis is immediate, the casualty will be unable to use his arms or legs to swim to safety and will lie limply in the water.

c. More often he will surface complaining of severe pain in his neck, back, arms or legs.

d. Ask the casualty if he has any unusual sensations such as numbness, burning or tingling in his hands or feet.

e. See if he is able to move all four limbs.

f. If you have **any** suspicion that a spinal injury may have occurred treat the casualty as if it has.

● RESCUE

To handle a casualty with a spinal injury correctly requires **at least** two rescuers if at all possible. It is important to bring the casualty to safety whilst protecting his spinal cord. Immobilisation in shallow water and on land is essential, and should be continued until the injured person receives medical attention. A special board for the rescue of such casualties may be available, but if not, try and find something suitable such as a wide plank of wood, a surf board etc. Before removing him from the water, secure the casualty on the board, maintaining alignment of his head, spine and feet. Alternatively support his head in your hands.

If the casualty with a fractured spine is moved roughly or any more than is absolutely necessary, permanent paralysis may result, even though it was not present at the time of the injury. If the casualty is unconscious and a spinal injury is suspected, treat him as if his neck were broken.

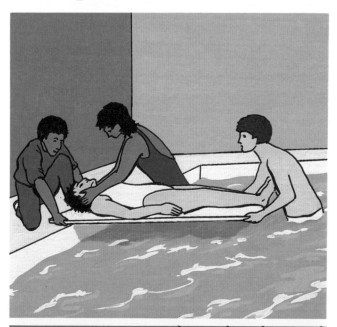

● RESUSCITATION

1. Immobilise the casualty on some form of board if available.
2. If breathing is absent or noisy, clear the airway by checking quickly for debris or loose false teeth in his mouth. Then lift his jaw **without** extending his neck, at the same time pressing down on his forehead with your other hand to steady his head.
3. If this does not result in the return of normal breathing start Expired Air Resuscitation by the mouth-to-mouth technique.
4. If you are unable to blow air in to the casualty's lungs because of an obstructed airway, carefully extend his neck bit by bit, attempting EAR after each additional amount of extension.
5. Check the carotid pulse. If it is absent, combine External Chest Compression with EAR in the usual way (see Chapter 3).
6. When breathing returns, leave the casualty on his back even if he remains unconscious. Maintain jaw lift at the same time as keeping his head still and in line with the rest of his body.
7. Medical attention should be obtained as a matter of considerable urgency.

Successful resuscitation that results in paralysis because the neck has been extended is a tragedy, but failure to carry out adequate resuscitation when breathing has stopped will result in certain death.

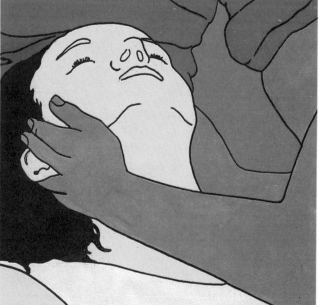

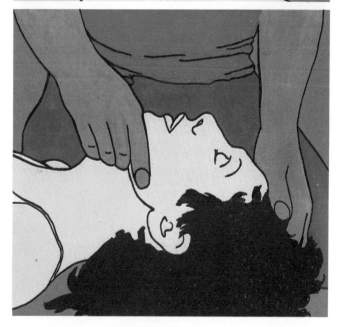

Epilepsy

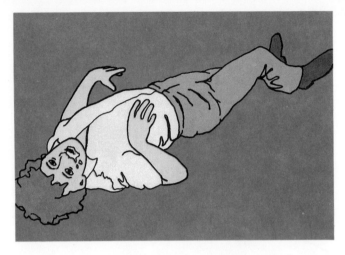

Introduction

Epilepsy is a condition in which sudden abnormal electrical discharges occur in the brain. Classically this produces a Major Fit ("Grand Mal" or convulsion) in which the sufferer becomes unconscious, falls to the ground and makes involuntary movements which can be quite violent. Because breathing is interfered with, cyanosis may develop and froth may appear at the mouth. After the attack the sufferer is often confused or sleepy for a while. There are milder forms of epilepsy, such as Psychomotor Attacks which occur when only a portion of the brain is affected by the abnormal electrical discharge. In these cases there may be involuntary movements such as twitching, plucking at clothing or lip smacking. The person appears conscious, but may be unable to speak or respond during the attack. Minor Attacks ("Petit Mal" or absences) may pass unnoticed, the person appearing merely to day-dream or stare blankly.

The advice of the British Epilepsy Association is that a person known to suffer from epilepsy should be allowed to swim provided:

a. He has approval from his own doctor.

b. He is accompanied by a strong swimmer, preferably a qualified Lifesaver, who is in the water with him.

c. He and his companion are both watched by a third person on the poolside.

Surprisingly few attacks occur whilst swimming, but a minimum water temperature of 26°C is recommended.

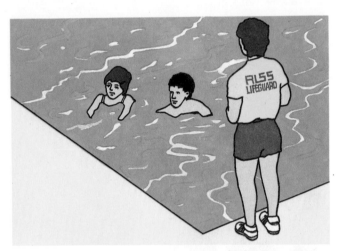

● TREATMENT
On Dry Land

1. A person having a Psychomotor or Minor Attack may well not require any attention except understanding.

2. During a Major Attack do not restrain the casualty and only move him if he is in danger of injuring himself or falling into the water.

3. Remove any objects which he may hit.

4. Do not try to put anything hard between his teeth as this can cause injury.

5. After the fit is over, allow him to rest with something soft under his head until he fully recovers.

6. Do not call an ambulance or doctor unless the casualty is injured, the attack lasts more than 15 minutes or is repeated without consciousness being regained in between times.

In The Water

1. After a Minor Attack help the casualty quietly and calmly out of the pool.

2. During a Major Attack keep the casualty's face above water, either by holding his head or lifting him under his arms from behind. Be careful not to allow his head to hit you.

3. If possible, tow him to shallow water and continue supporting his head until the attack is over.

4. Remove him from the pool with an assistant as soon as the abnormal movements cease.

5. Be prepared to start Expired Air Resuscitation if breathing does not restart.

6. If there is any possibility that he may have inhaled water or if resuscitation has been necessary, make certain that he receives medical attention.

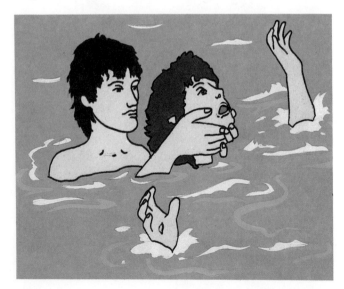

Effects of Heat

Introduction

People involved in sport and recreation by the seaside or other open water may suffer the effects of excessive exposure to sunlight and heat. A Lifeguard patrol in particular, may be called upon to deal with cases of heat exhaustion, heatstroke or sunburn.

Heat Exhaustion

This is caused by loss of salt and water from the body due to excessive sweating. It is seen particularly after prolonged exercise in hot, humid weather. It is more likely to occur if the casualty has not been drinking adequate amounts of fluid.

● DIAGNOSIS

a. The casualty may complain of feeling exhausted, tired, dizzy or sick, but as some degree of mental confusion is common, he may be unaware of his condition.
b. He may complain or indicate that he has muscle cramps in the legs and abdomen.
c. The signs of shock may be present (see page 9), the casualty appearing pale, with a cold clammy skin, rapid breathing and a rapid weak pulse.

● TREATMENT

1. Rest the casualty in a cool place.
2. If he is conscious give him **sips** of cool water. If he is sweating profusely or complains of muscle cramp add small quantities of salt – half a teaspoon to one pint (half a litre) of water.
3. If the casualty becomes unconscious, is very drowsy, or has any difficulty swallowing, do not attempt to give any further fluids but put him in the Recovery Position (see page 26).
4. Obtain medical assistance urgently if there is any impairment of consciousness.
5. **Only** if you are sure that the cause of shock is overheating and sweating should fluids be given by mouth.

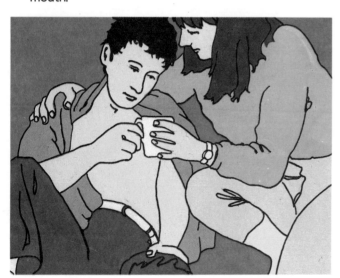

Heat Stroke

This condition may be produced by a very hot environment or by prolonged exposure to the sun. Whereas in heat exhaustion the problem is that the body loses salt and water through sweating, in heat stroke the casualty becomes unable to prevent his body temperature rising so that it may reach 40°C (104°F) or more. Although rare, it is a serious condition which can rapidly lead to unconsciousness and death.

● DIAGNOSIS

a. The casualty complains of headache, weakness and feeling hot.
b. He may be restless or may rapidly become unconscious.
c. He will feel hot to the touch and be flushed, although the skin remains dry.
d. The pulse is rapid but feels "full" and bounding.

● TREATMENT

1. Lay the casualty down in a cool place with his head supported.
2. Reduce his body temperature by wrapping him in cold wet towels or sheets, or by fanning him with paper or an electric fan if available.
3. If he becomes unconscious, check his breathing and institute Expired Air Resuscitation (see page 20), as required. If his breathing is normal place him in the Recovery Position (see page 26).
4. Summon medical aid (ambulance) as a matter of considerable urgency.

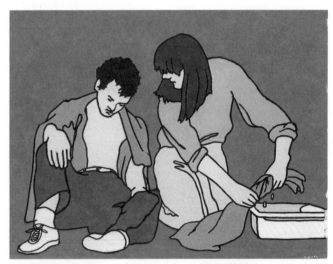

Sunburn

Prolonged exposure to the sun can result in burning of the skin, which may not be apparent to the casualty until the damage has been done. Windy conditions make burning more likely as does a skin wet from sea or sweat.

● TREATMENT

1. Remove the casualty to shade.
2. Cool the affected parts by sponging with cold water.
3. Do not break any blisters, but cover raw areas with a clean cloth or other dressing.
4. If the burning is extensive or the casualty shows any signs of shock, medical attention should be sought.

For the effects of cold, see Chapter 6.

Asthma

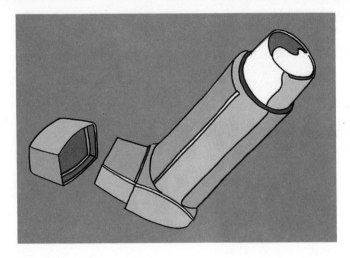

Introduction

The walls of the bronchi (air passages) inside the chest contain muscle. In some people this muscle may go into spasm, either during exercise or because dust or pollen to which the person is allergic has been inhaled. The result is narrowing of the bronchi and interference with breathing, so that the casualty becomes short of breath and wheezy. This condition is known as asthma.

Typically, the sufferer is quite well between the attacks which may come on very suddenly and pass off again just as quickly. Probably because the air above the surface of the swimming pool is moist, asthma is less likely to occur during swimming than during other forms of exercise. For this reason asthmatics are often encouraged to take up swimming, although if their attacks are severe, it is advisable for some form of supervision to be available.

● PREVENTION OF ATTACKS

1. Sufferers from asthma often carry a special aerosol (spray) with them and their doctor may advise them to take a "puff" just before going swimming.
2. Anxiety may bring on an attack, so the swimming or lifesaving teacher should adopt a particularly calm approach towards the weak or non-swimmer.
3. If the sufferer is already wheezy, do not allow him to swim, unless use of his medication relieves his breathing difficulties.

● DIAGNOSIS OF AN ATTACK

a. The casualty may be very anxious.
b. Breathing is obviously difficult and noisy, the wheeze being heard particularly on expiration (breathing out).

● TREATMENT

1. Reassure the casualty.
2. Help him out of the water.
3. Sit him down, preferably on a chair leaning **slightly** forward.
4. Find his medication or aerosol and allow him to use it.
5. If the attack is mild and rapidly relieved, allow him to return to the pool, but observe him for any recurrence.
6. If the attack is severe or unrelieved in a few minutes by his medication, or if the casualty becomes very distressed, obtain medical assistance.

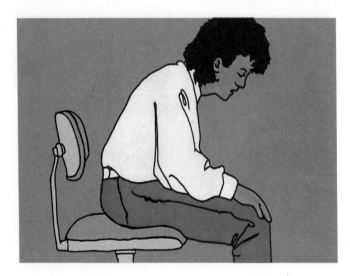

Chapter 6
The Effects of Cold Water Immersion

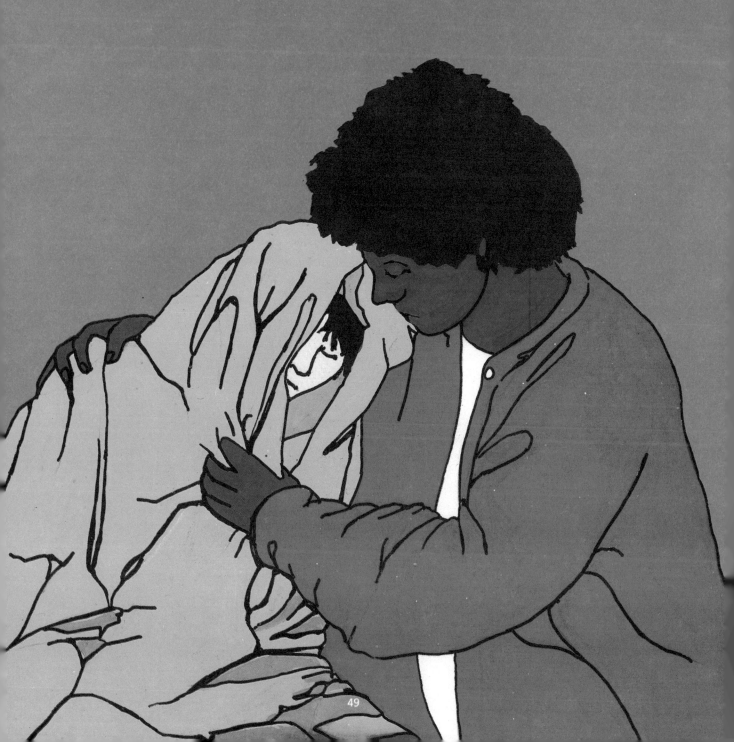

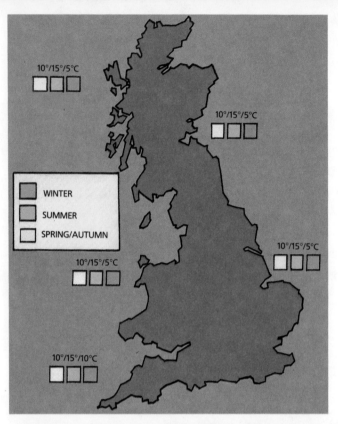

10°/15°/5°C ☐☐☐

10°/15°/5°C ☐☐☐

☐ WINTER
☐ SUMMER
☐ SPRING/AUTUMN

10°/15°/5°C ☐☐☐

10°/15°/5°C ☐☐☐

10°/15°/10°C ☐☐☐

Introduction

Most people in the United Kingdom learn to swim in heated pools and never experience the effects of cold water; on the other hand most drownings occur in rivers, lakes and the sea, where the water temperature is very low. Around the British coast the sea temperature rarely rises above 15°C and in winter it falls to 5°C or below.

Cold water immersion is probably the main cause of death from drowning in Britain at any time of the year. Even when asphyxia due to submersion is the predominant problem, a damaging degree of chilling is often present as well. The effects of cold water on the body can be considered under the following headings:

- Sudden entry into cold water
- Cold water and swimming ability
- Prolonged immersion in cold water

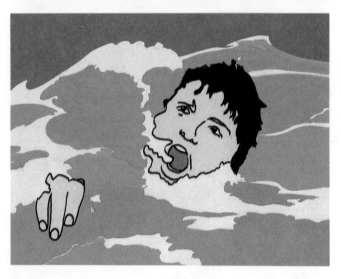

Sudden entry into cold water

As anyone who has taken a cold shower will know, sudden exposure to cold water (around 15°C) "takes your breath away." The effect is to produce an uncontrollable gasping which lasts for a minute or so. The increased rate and depth of breathing is considerably greater than the body requires, with the result that the level of carbon dioxide in the blood falls. This can lead to dizziness or even loss of consciousness which incapacitates the sufferer. In addition, if breath is drawn-in whilst the casualty is submerged or a wave is breaking over his face, he may inhale water.

Immersion in cold water affects blood pressure and pulse rate, causing both to rise. In the young fit person this is of no consequence, but in the older casualty or one who has pre-existing heart or circulatory disease it can result in a heart attack or stroke.

In a few otherwise fit people sudden immersion may produce cardiac arrest. It is thought that this is due to a nervous reflex occurring when cold water strikes the face.

Swimming in cold water

In very cold water (around 5°C), even strong swimmers are unable to keep afloat for more than a few minutes, after which they suddenly fail and sink. This failure is believed to be due to the rapid breathing brought about by the cold and the difficulty experienced in co-ordinating breaths with swimming. In addition, more effort is required to swim in cold water due to its increased viscosity.

Prolonged cold immersion

Human beings, like other mammals, require a near-constant body temperature in order to function normally. For man, the central core of the body needs to remain very near to 37°C. If body temperature rises in hot weather, blood is directed to the skin surface. Sweating occurs, and heat is drawn from the body as the sweat evaporates. On the other hand, in cold conditions blood is withdrawn from the surface to minimise loss of heat, and shivering generates extra heat from muscle activity.

If body temperature falls to 35°C or below, the casualty is by definition suffering from hypothermia. As the temperature falls further the casualty becomes confused, gradually loses consciousness, and breathing becomes more difficult and sometimes wheezy. The heart beats more slowly and then irregularly. By the time the casualty's temperature has reached 30°C he is usually unconscious, and if it falls much further he dies.

The rate at which a person cools depends upon the temperature of the water in which he is immersed, how fat he is, what clothes he is wearing and what movements he makes.

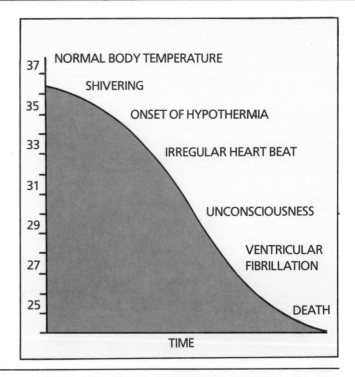

Body fat

Body fat acts as insulation and the length of time a person can survive in the cold is directly related to his fatness, as measured by skin-fold thickness. For example, small thin children, who have a large surface area in relation to their size, can cool to hypothermic levels within 30 minutes if immersed in water at 20°C. In contrast, very fat adults can maintain their body temperatures in near-freezing water for an hour or more.

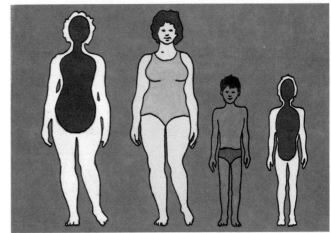

Clothing

Even light and non-waterproof clothing can substantially reduce heat loss by preventing the continuous movement of cold water around the body. Out of the water, clothing also helps to prevent "wind chill" which aggravates heat loss, particularly if the parts exposed are wet. Ideally, clothing worn when at risk of immersion, for example when sailing, should be fully waterproof. The head should be covered as this is an area from which much heat is lost.

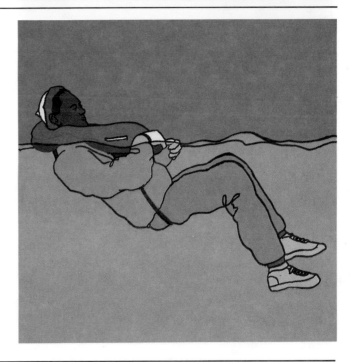

Hypothermia

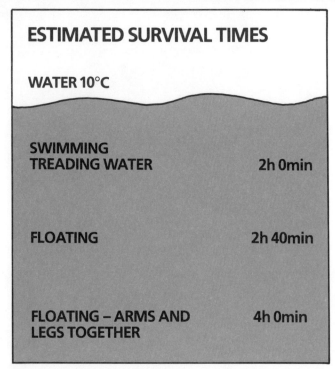

ESTIMATED SURVIVAL TIMES

WATER 10°C

SWIMMING TREADING WATER	2h 0min
FLOATING	2h 40min
FLOATING – ARMS AND LEGS TOGETHER	4h 0min

Activity

The natural tendency when feeling cold is to move around. This is logical in that muscle activity produces heat. Exercise however, also results in a greater flow of blood to the muscles and to the skin surface. In water below about 20°C the loss of heat from blood at the body surface becomes greater than the gain of heat from exercise. It has been shown that in cold water the time taken for the body temperature to fall (and hypothermia to occur) is considerably longer if the casualty floats motionless with legs together and elbows to the sides (the HELP position) rather than swims around. Obviously this can only be achieved if a buoyancy aid is worn.

Alcohol and hypothermia

If alcohol is consumed even in small quantities (one or two measures of spirits or their equivalent) and the drinker then undertakes exercise, there can be a substantial fall in the level of sugar in the blood. This can lead to mental confusion and a rapid drop in body temperature. Swimming, particularly in cold water, after having taken alcohol is extremely dangerous. Recent statistics have shown that in up to 25 per cent of all drownings, alcohol consumption is a contributory factor.

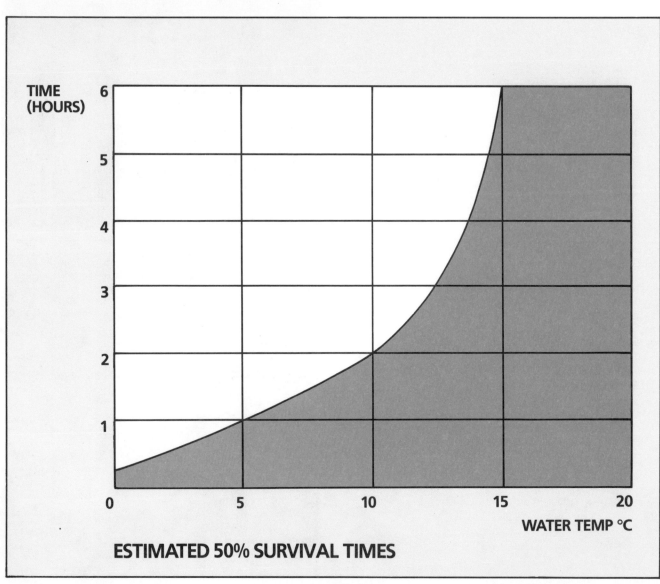

ESTIMATED 50% SURVIVAL TIMES

Avoiding the dangers of cold water immersion

1. If intentionally swimming

a. Be aware of the differences between swimming in warm and cold water.

b. Never make a sudden entry into cold water; be particularly careful if you are over the age of 35 years or are known to have any heart or circulatory disease.

c. Do not over-estimate your swimming ability, which is considerably reduced in cold water. Stay within your depth.

d. Never drink alcohol before swimming.

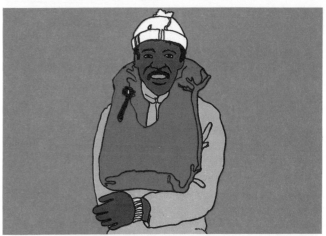

2. If in danger of unintentional immersion

a. Before going out in any boat liable to capsize, or if imminent immersion is anticipated, put on several layers of warm clothing, preferably with a waterproof suit on top. Wear an efficient life jacket. If possible also wear gloves and socks and cover your head.

b. On sudden entry into cold water, do not panic, but hold on to a support or float quietly, facing away from the waves, until the initial distress is over.

c. Do not swim unless you are forced to do so to keep afloat or to get clear of danger.

d. Do not try to swim for the shore unless this is within a short distance – 200 metres in cold water; 50 metres in very cold water.

e. Do not move more than is absolutely necessary; do not attempt to exercise to keep warm.

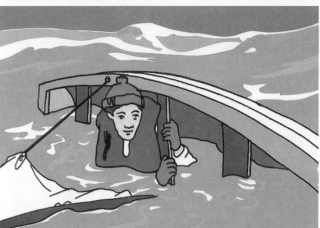

f. Do not remove clothing, except items which interfere with flotation (heavy overcoats; boots).

g. Try and keep your head above water. Intermittent submersion of the head will increase heat loss.

h. Face away from waves to prevent water splashing your face.

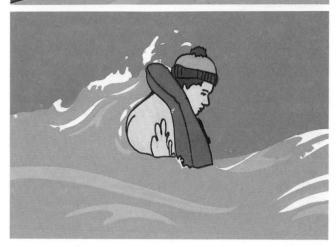

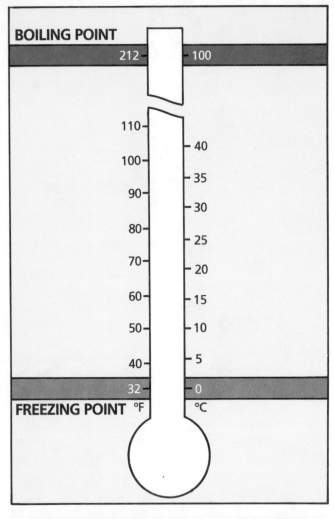

BOILING POINT

°F	°C
212	100
110	40
100	35
90	30
80	25
70	20
60	15
50	10
40	5
32	0

FREEZING POINT °F °C

● DIAGNOSIS

The possibility of hypothermia should always be kept in mind when dealing with casualties rescued from the water even if it does not appear to be particularly cold. Confirmation is difficult without a special low-reading thermometer, but consider the diagnosis if the casualty has suffered prolonged immersion, is a child or elderly person, or if the water conditions are particularly bad.

a. The casualty will feel and look cold.

b. Shivering will be present if hypothermia is mild, but in severe cases it is often absent.

c. There may be mental confusion or even unconsciousness.

d. Breathing may be laboured or noisy.

e. The pulse may be difficult or impossible to feel. If present, it may be weak and irregular.

● TREATMENT

When the heart cools below 30°C it becomes irritable and liable to develop ventricular fibrillation (one form of cardiac arrest). A particularly vulnerable period is the first few minutes after a casualty is removed from cold water, when any rough handling may precipitate ventricular fibrillation.

1. Remove casualty from the water keeping him as horizontal as possible.

2. Handle him gently and avoid sudden or jolting movements.

3. Check adequacy of breathing and presence of carotid pulse, instituting resuscitation (CPR) as necessary (See Chapter 3).

4. Provide a shelter away from wind and rain. If necessary, carefully move the casualty a short distance, but only after any resuscitation has been successfully undertaken.

5. Only if the casualty is conscious, has been completely removed from exposure to the cold, and dry clothing or other covering is available, should his wet clothes be removed. This should be carried out as quickly and as gently as possible by at least two rescuers.

6. Warm the casualty by wrapping him in dry blankets, towels or available clothing, remembering to cover his head and limbs as well as his trunk.

7. Never apply local heat (hot water bottle; massage etc.) as this provides little warmth for the body, but encourages blood to move to the surface, with consequent loss of body heat and a possible detrimental lowering of blood pressure.

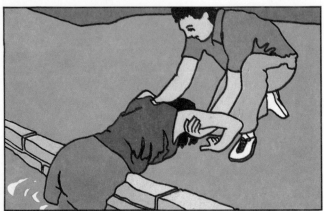

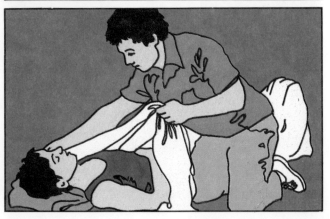

8. If a bath or shower is available, this can be used for the casualty with mild hypothermia (fully conscious and shivering):
    - Water should be 40°C (hand hot).
    - Fully immerse the casualty (except for his head) into deep water in order to exert a "squeeze" on his body. This prevents a fall in blood pressure which can occur as the blood vessels near the skin surface relax.
    - If a shower is used the casualty should sit or squat.
9. Urgent medical attention should be obtained, usually by summoning an ambulance:
    - If any resuscitation has been necessary.
    - If the casualty has been unconscious, even for a short time.
    - If prolonged (more than a few minutes) involuntary immersion has occured.
10. In all other cases, especially if inhalation of water is suspected, less urgent medical advice should be sought. The exception is when the casualty has remained fully conscious and rational, has been shivering throughout the incident, and has fully recovered after rewarming.

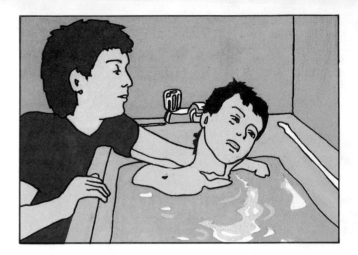

● NOTES

A number of cases have been reported in medical literature in which resuscitation has been successful in casualties who have been completely submerged for periods of 30-40 minutes in very cold water. A mechanism of survival, akin to that which allows aquatic mammals to stay underwater for a considerable length of time, has been postulated. Also reported, have been cases in which apparently dead victims of hypothermia have eventually recovered after more than an hour of resuscitation. The message is: Do not give up attempts at resuscitation too easily or too soon.

Glossary of Terms

Adam's Apple — A colloquial term for the cartilage which protects the larynx (voice box)

Airway — The passages by which air enters and leaves the lungs

Alveolus (pl. alveoli) — Tiny, thin-walled air sac in the lung.

Artery — A vessel (tube) which takes blood away from the heart

Asphyxia — Insufficient oxygen reaching the tissues of the body

Asystole — Complete inactivity of the ventricles of the heart

Atrium (pl. atria) — One of the two upper chambers of the heart

Bronchus (pl. bronchi) — Tube-like air passage in the lung

Capillary — A small, thin-walled blood vessel

Carbon dioxide (CO_2) — A gas, found in very small amounts in atmospheric air, but in higher concentration in expired air

Cardiac arrest — Cessation of heart beat

Cardiopulmonary Resuscitation (CPR) — Combined Expired Air Resuscitation (EAR) and External Chest Compression (EEC)

Carotid Artery — An artery running up the side of the neck

Cartilage — Gristle. Found, for example, in the nose, larynx and in joints.

Cilia — Tiny, hair-like structures which line the bronchi

Contract — Shorten (as of a muscle)

Diabetes — A disease in which the body is unable to handle sugar and other carbohydrates correctly

Diaphragm — A dome-shaped muscle which separates the chest from abdomen

Digestion — The process of breaking food down into a form in which it can be absorbed

Drowning — Death caused by asphyxia due to immersion in water

    Dry-drowning – Drowning in which no water reaches the lungs

    Near-drowning – Survival of a casualty after an immersion incident

    Secondary-drowning – Outpouring of fluid from the blood into the alveoli due to irritation by inhaled water

EAR — Expired Air Resuscitation

ECC — External Chest Compression

ECG — Electrocardiogram

Electro-cardiogram — A recording, usually on a paper strip, of the electrical activity of the heart

Epiglottis — A tongue-like flap of cartilage which prevents food entering the larynx

Epilepsy — A condition in which abnormal electrical discharges in the brain produce "fits"

Expiration — Breathing out

Expired Air Resuscitation — (Colloq. Kiss of Life) Blowing air into a casualty's mouth or nose to maintain life when breathing has stopped

First Aid — The initial or emergency help given to a casualty before qualified medical assistance is available

Fracture — A break in a bone

Heart Attack — Coronary thrombosis. Damage to the heart muscle due to interruption of its blood supply

Heart Failure — Failure of the heart to maintain an adequate circulation of blood

Hyperventilation — Deliberate or involuntary overbreathing

Hypothermia — Reduction of the deep body (core) temperature to 35°C or below

Inspiration — Breathing in

Larynx — That portion of the airway in the upper neck which contains the vocal cords. The voice box.

Oesophagus — A muscular tube which acts as a food passage through the chest from the mouth to the stomach. The gullet

Oxygen (O_2) — A gas, essential for life, which makes up about 21% of the air

Pharynx — Back of the mouth. Throat

Plasma — The fluid part of blood

Platelets — Small particles in the blood which are necessary for clotting to take place

Pneumonia — Inflammation of the lung, usually caused by an infection

Pulse — Impulse felt in an artery with each beat of the heart

Recovery Position — The position in which an unconscious casualty is placed to allow observation of his breathing and prevent obstruction of the airway

Red Blood Cells Red Blood Corpuscles — Those cells in the blood which carry oxygen

Respiration — 1. Breathing 2. The complete process of getting oxygen to the cells of the body and getting rid of carbon dioxide

Respiratory Centre — The part of the brain which controls the rate and depth of breathing

Resuscitation — The act of reviving a nearly dead or apparently dead casualty

Shock — Failure of the circulation which results in an inadequate supply of blood to vital organs

Skeleton — The framework of bones which supports the body and protects the internal organs

Spinal Cord — The column of nerve tissue, continuous with the base of the brain, which is protected by the bony spine

Sputum — Mucus coughed-up from the bronchi

Sternum — The flat bone, lying in the front of the chest, to which most of the ribs are attached

Stroke — Damage to the brain due to an interruption of part of its blood supply

Suffocation — Obstruction of the airway, preventing an adequate amount of air reaching the lungs

Thorax — The chest

Trachea — The semi-rigid tube, felt in the front of the neck, that takes air from the larynx into the chest

Vein — A vessel (tube) which takes blood back to the heart

Vena Cava (pl. Venae Cavae) — Major vein that brings blood back to the heart from the upper (superior vena cava) and lower (inferior vena cava) parts of the body

Ventricle — One of the two lower chambers of the heart

Ventricular Fibrillation — Irregular, ineffective twitching of the ventricles of the heart which produces no circulation of blood